MW01223413

Chronic Fatigue Syndrome: Critical Reviews and Clinical Advances

Chronic Fatigue Syndrome: Critical Reviews and Clinical Advances has been co-published simultaneously as *Journal of Chronic Fatigue Syndrome*, Volume 6, Numbers 3/4 2000.

The *Journal of Chronic Fatigue Syndrome* Monographic "Separates"

Below is a list of "separates," which in serials librarianship means a special issue simultaneously published as a special journal issue or double-issue *and* as a "separate" hardbound monograph. (This is a format which we also call a "DocuSerial.")

"Separates" are published because specialized libraries or professionals may wish to purchase a specific thematic issue by itself in a format which can be separately cataloged and shelved, as opposed to purchasing the journal on an on-going basis. Faculty members may also more easily consider a "separate" for classroom adoption.

"Separates" are carefully classified separately with the major book jobbers so that the journal tie-in can be noted on new book order slips to avoid duplicate purchasing.

You may wish to visit Haworth's website at . . .

http://www.haworthpressinc.com

. . . to search our online catalog for complete tables of contents of these separates and related publications.

You may also call 1-800-HAWORTH (outside US/Canada: 607-722-5857), or Fax 1-800-895-0582 (outside US/Canada: 607-771-0012), or e-mail at:

getinfo@haworthpressinc.com

Chronic Fatigue Syndrome: Critical Reviews and Clinical Advances, edited by Kenny De Meirleir, MD, PhD, and Roberto Patarca-Montero, MD, PhD (Vol. 6, No. 3/4, 2000). *The reviews in this volume provide the specialized views of different schools of thought, research, and clinical intervention for CFS and ME (myalgic encephalomyelitis). Edited by the organizer of the Second World Congress on Chronic Fatigue Syndrome and Related Disorders, this work focuses on information gathered there. Keep your knowledge of these disorders current and up-to-date with Chronic Fatigue Syndrome: Critical Reviews and Clinical Advances!*

Chronic Fatigue Syndrome: Advances in Epidemiologic, Clinical, and Basic Science Research, edited by Roberto Patarca-Montero, MD, PhD (Vol. 5, No. 3/4, 1999). *Highlights the presentations and issues discussed at the recent Fourth Annual International Conference of the American Association of Chronic Fatigue Syndrome (CFS). You will explore the strengths and weaknesses of current case definitions of CFS and how these can be improved. Also, you will examine how to distinguish CFS from other similar ailments such as fibromyalgia and multiple chemical sensitivity. This book puts different therapeutic modalities to the test, and addresses the neurological and psychiatric manifestations associated with CFS.*

Disability and Chronic Fatigue Syndrome: Clinical, Legal and Patient Perspectives, edited by Nancy G. Klimas, MD, and Roberto Patarca, MD, PhD (Vol. 3, No. 4, 1997). *"As a physician who deals with disability issues daily, I found this volume fascinating and informative. This is 'must read' material for anyone involved with the disability process and CFS." (Charles W. Lapp, MD, Director, Hunter-Hopkins Center, Charlotte, North Carolina)*

Clinical Management of Chronic Fatigue Syndrome: Clinical Conference, American Association of Chronic Fatigue Syndrome, edited by Nancy Klimas, MD, and Roberto Patarca, MD, PhD (Vol. 1, No. 3/4, 1995). *"A truly interdisciplinary approach to the investigation and management of a debilitating and complex disorder." (The Annals of Pharmacotherapy)*

Chronic Fatigue Syndrome: Critical Reviews and Clinical Advances

Kenny De Meirleir, MD, PhD
Roberto Patarca-Montero, MD, PhD
Editors

Chronic Fatigue Syndrome: Critical Reviews and Clinical Advances has been co-published simultaneously as *Journal of Chronic Fatigue Syndrome*, Volume 6, Numbers 3/4 2000.

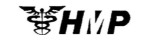

The Haworth Medical Press
An Imprint of
The Haworth Press, Inc.
New York • London • Oxford

Published by

The Haworth Medical Press®, 10 Alice Street, Binghamton, NY 13904-1580 USA

The Haworth Medical Press® is an imprint of The Haworth Press, Inc., 10 Alice Street, Binghamton, NY 13904-1580 USA.

Chronic Fatigue Syndrome: Critical Reviews and Clinical Advances has been co-published simultaneously as *Journal of Chronic Fatigue Syndrome*, Volume 6, Numbers 3/4 2000.

The development, preparation, and publication of this work has been undertaken with great care. However, the publisher, employees, editors, and agents of The Haworth Press and all imprints of The Haworth Press, Inc., including The Haworth Medical Press® and Pharmaceutical Products Press®, are not responsible for any errors contained herein or for consequences that may ensue from use of materials or information contained in this work. Opinions expressed by the author(s) are not necessarily those of The Haworth Press, Inc.

Cover design by Thomas J. Mayshock Jr.

Library of Congress Cataloging-in-Publication Data

Chronic fatigue syndrome: critical reviews and clinical advances/Kenny De Meirleir, Roberto Patarca-Montero, editors.
      p.; cm.–(Journal of chronic fatigue syndrome; v.6, no. 3/4)
      Includes bibliographical references and index.
      ISBN 0-7890-0998-6 (alk. paper)–ISBN 0-7890-0999-4 (alk. paper)
      1. Chronic fatigue syndrome. I. Meirleir, K. De (Kenny) II. Patarca-Montero, Roberto III. Series.
      [DNLM: 1. Fatigue Syndrome, Chronic. WB 146 C55663 2000]
RB150.F37 C48 2000
616'.0478–dc21
                                   00-056714

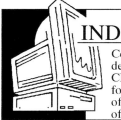

INDEXING & ABSTRACTING

Contributions to this publication are selectively indexed or abstracted in print, electronic, online, or CD-ROM version(s) of the reference tools and information services listed below. This list is current as of the copyright date of this publication. See the end of this section for additional notes.

- *Abstracts in Anthropology*
- *Abstracts of Research in Pastoral Care & Counseling*
- *AIDS Abstracts*
- *Behavioral Medicine Abstracts*
- *BUBL Information Service, an Internet-Based Information Service for the UK higher education community, <URL: http://bubl.ac.uk/>*
- *Centre Regional d'Exploration des Myalgias*
- *CFS-NEWS*
- *CINAHL (Cumulative Index to Nursing & Allied Health Literature)*
- *CNPIEC Reference Guide: Chinese National Directory of Foreign Periodicals*
- *Digest of Neurology and Psychiatry*
- *EMBASE/Excerpta Medica Secondary Publishing Division*
- *FINDEX www.publist.com*
- *Greenfiles*
- *Human Resources Abstracts (HRA)*
- *Industrial Hygiene Digest*
- *Journal of College Science Teaching (abstracts section)*
- *Leeds Medical Information*
- *MANTIS (Manual, Alternative & Natural Therapy)*
- *ME and CFS Capita Selecta Quarterly, UK*
- *Mental Health Abstracts (online through DIALOG)*
- *National Library of Medicine "Abstracts Section"*
- *Nutrition Research Newsletter "Abstracts Section"*
- *PASCAL, c/o Institute de L'Information Scientifique et Technique*
- *Pediatric Pain Letter*

(continued)

- *Pharmacist's Letter "Abstracts Section"*
- *Published International Literature on Traumatic Stress (The PILOTS Database)*
- *Referativnyi Zhurnal (Abstracts Journal of the All-Russian Institute of Scientific and Technical Information)*
- *REHABDATA, National Rehabilitation Information Center*
- *Sapient Health Network*
- *Selected Abstracts on Occupational Diseases (DHSSDATA)*
- *Social Services Abstracts*
- *Sociological Abstracts (SA)*
- *Violence and Abuse Abstracts: A Review of Current Literature on Interpersonal Violence (VAA)*

Special Bibliographic Notes related to special journal issues (separates) and indexing/abstracting:

- indexing/abstracting services in this list will also cover material in any "separate" that is co-published simultaneously with Haworth's special thematic journal issue or DocuSerial. Indexing/abstracting usually covers material at the article/chapter level.
- monographic co-editions are intended for either non-subscribers or libraries which intend to purchase a second copy for their circulating collections.
- monographic co-editions are reported to all jobbers/wholesalers/approval plans. The source journal is listed as the "series" to assist the prevention of duplicate purchasing in the same manner utilized for books-in-series.
- to facilitate user/access services all indexing/abstracting services are encouraged to utilize the co-indexing entry note indicated at the bottom of the first page of each article/chapter/contribution.
- this is intended to assist a library user of any reference tool (whether print, electronic, online, or CD-ROM) to locate the monographic version if the library has purchased this version but not a subscription to the source journal.
- individual articles/chapters in any Haworth publication are also available through the Haworth Document Delivery Service (HDDS).

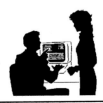

Chronic Fatigue Syndrome:
Critical Reviews and Clinical Advances

CONTENTS

ABOUT THE EDITORS

Kenny De Meirleir, MD, PhD, is Professor of Physiology and Medicine at the Vrije Universiteit Brussel, where he is Director of the Human Performance Laboratory (BLITS) and Member of "the Vakgroep" Internal Medicine. His interest in Chronic Fatigue Syndrome dates back to 1989. Dr. K. De Meirleir serves on the Board of Directors of several non-profit scientific organisations and is member of the Editorial Board of the *Journal of Chronic Fatigue Syndrome.*

He has co-authored numerous journal articles and book chapters on different subjects. Through lectures and support of patients groups, he tries to increase awareness of CFS in Europe.

Roberto Patarca-Montero, MD, PhD, is Assistant Professor of Medicine and Microbiology and Immunology and also serves as Director of the E.M. Papper Laboratory of Clinical Immunology at the University of Miami, School of Medicine. Previously, he was Assistant Professor of Pathology at the Dana-Farber Cancer Institute and Harvard Medical School in Boston. Dr. Patarca-Montero is a member of the Board of Directors of the American Association for Chronic Fatigue Syndrome. Dr. Patarca-Montero also serves as editor of *Critical Reviews in Oncogenesis* and is the author or co-author of more than 100 articles in journals or books. He is currently conducting research on immunotherapy in AIDS and chronic fatigue syndrome.

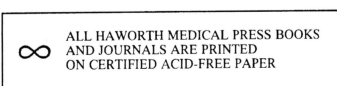

Introduction

Kenny De Meirleir, MD, PhD
Roberto Patarca-Montero, MD, PhD

The reviews in this publication provide the specialized views of different schools of thought, research and clinical intervention for chronic fatigue syndrome and myalgic encephalomyelitis (CFS/ME). This apparently divergent specialization trend is providing very important information on particular subpopulations of patients. For instance, some patients present with a clear picture of immune activation while in others autonomic dysfunction is the predominant disorder. As we deepen our vertical knowledge of particular clinical presentations that recruit the talents and experience of diverse specialists, we may start to find unifying principles with more solid holding, a process that may allow the pinpointing of a common etiology to become a reality. The evolution of the study of CFS/ME has witnessed several inductive-deductive cycles, each one increasing our knowledge base and creating more effective therapeutic approaches for particular symptomatologies. We may find that, even if we decipher the common etiopathological denominator, the pharmacological and therapeutic armamentarium available may not be effective for the treatment of CFS/ME as is the case for the treatment of many infectious, neurological or autoimmune diseases. We are pleased to continue to provide a scholarly forum for these challenging ailments and to bring sound research, hypotheses, reviews, and preliminary clinical reports to expanding professional and lay audiences. Dr. Rosamund Vallings wrote a report for this issue on the highlights of the Second World Congress on Chronic Fatigue Syndrome and Related Disorders.

[Haworth co-indexing entry note]: "Introduction." De Meirleir, Kenny and Roberto Patarca-Montero. Co-published simultaneously in *Journal of Chronic Fatigue Syndrome* (The Haworth Medical Press, an imprint of The Haworth Press, Inc.) Vol. 6, No. 3/4, 2000, p. 1; and: *Chronic Fatigue Syndrome: Critical Reviews and Clinical Advances* (ed: Kenny De Meirleir, and Roberto Patarca-Montero) The Haworth Medical Press, an imprint of The Haworth Press, Inc., 2000, p. 1. Single or multiple copies of this article are available for a fee from The Haworth Document Delivery Service [1-800-342-9678, 9:00 a.m. - 5:00 p.m. (EST). E-mail address: getinfo@haworthpressinc.com].

CRITICAL REVIEWS

Report on the Second World Congress on Chronic Fatigue Syndrome and Related Disorders: Towards Effective Diagnosis and Treatment in the 21st Century

Rosamund Vallings, MB BS

From 9-12 September, 1999, I was privileged to attend the Second World Congress on Chronic Fatigue Syndrome and Related Disorders. This was hosted and efficiently organised by Professor Kenny De Meirleir and his team from the Vrije Universiteit Brussels. On the first afternoon we attended a pre-conference symposium on Gulf War Illness. Then followed 2 intensive days of presentations of scientific papers coupled with posters displaying a wide range of scientific

Rosamund Vallings is affiliated with the University of Auckland, 140 North Road, Papakura, New Zealand (E-mail: Vallings@xtra.co.nz).

[Haworth co-indexing entry note]: "Report on the Second World Congress on Chronic Fatigue Syndrome and Related Disorders: Towards Effective Diagnosis and Treatment in the 21st Century." Vallings, Rosamund. Co-published simultaneously in *Journal of Chronic Fatigue Syndrome* (The Haworth Medical Press, an imprint of The Haworth Press, Inc.) Vol. 6, No. 3/4, 2000, pp. 3-21; and: *Chronic Fatigue Syndrome: Critical Reviews and Clinical Advances* (ed: Kenny De Meirleir, and Roberto Patarca-Montero) The Haworth Medical Press, an imprint of The Haworth Press, Inc., 2000, pp. 3-21. Single or multiple copies of this article are available for a fee from The Haworth Document Delivery Service [1-800-342-9678, 9:00 a.m. - 5:00 p.m. (EST). E-mail address: getinfo@haworthpressinc.com].

endeavour and new ideas. The conference was well attended by physicians, researchers, health workers and patients from all around the globe. There was ample opportunity for mixing and mingling at the regularly scheduled breaks, and as always this is the time for sharing of ideas and networking for future interaction. We were also treated to a relaxing social programme coupled with wonderful weather in which to enjoy Brussels at its best.

In the following report I have tried to follow the conference format, when the sessions were categorised according to various disciplines.

BIOCHEMISTRY

The conference opened with a keynote address by Neil McGregor, from Newcastle, Australia, who gave an overview of the current biochemical research in Australia, followed by a discussion of the biochemistry of chronic pain and fatigue. In their studies, no single virus has been implicated in Chronic Fatigue Syndrome (CFS) and 75% of patients, compared to 14% of controls, showed elevated RnaseL activity. The metabolic events associated with chronic pain differ from those associated with chronic fatigue. Chronic pain was associated with reductions in serum sodium, changes in urinary volume and output of amino and organic acids, increases in levels of markers of tissue damage (ALT, AST), and increase in the tyrosine/leucine ratio, representing alterations in protein turnover. Chronic fatigue was associated with alterations in urinary excretion of amino and organic acids associated with the tricarboxylic acid cycle.

Symptom expression relates to cytokine activity, urine volume and chemistry. The mechanism for chronic pain was clarified as related to catabolism (enhanced proteolysis) in muscles. We take amino acids from muscles as we fight infection and this leads to muscle protein depletion. A number of the urinary metabolites are altered in CFS, which provide evidence for proteolysis.

The urinary volume is increased in pain and fatigue states, and this can lead to reduced blood pressure and blood volume, coupled with loss of metabolites. This phenomenon is helped by added salt in the diet and the use of blood pressure raising medication. Antidepressants are found to be helpful by improving kidney function leading to reduction in urinary output, improved metabolism and reduction in fatigue.

McGregor then talked about myofascial pain, which occurs in 60-70% of CFS patients. Intensity of symptoms was found to correlate with carriage of toxin-producing coagulase negative staphylococci. This maybe a secondary contributory bacterial phenomenon. The presence of the toxin correlated positively with cytokine levels and symptom expression.

This discussion was furthered by Henry Butt, another of the Newcastle team. He discussed the association of the staphylococcal membrane-damaging toxin and chronic fatigue/pain. Ninety percent of 73 patients reviewed were found to be positive for the membrane-damaging toxin with almost nil being found in controls. Pain severity was found to correlate with level of toxin and significant alterations in urinary metabolites. In particular, tyrosine was elevated and leucine decreased signifying altered proteolysis. Cognitive function also correlated with toxin levels. It was recommended that nose, throat and low vaginal swabs should be taken when staph infection is suspected. If pain improves with antibiotic use, this may help confirm diagnosis.

Hugh Dunstan, Newcastle, then discussed the development of laboratory-based tests in relation to essential fatty acids (EFAs) and cholesterol. He reiterated the heterogeneity of CFS and the fact that we may never therefore have a yes/no definitive test for CFS *per se*. His research has shown that CFS patients had significantly different profiles of fatty acids and sterols compared with controls. The most important factors in discriminating controls from CFS patients were decreased elaidic acid and increased stearic acid. CFS patients also had low levels of cholesterol, which affects cell membrane integrity and function, steroid hormone synthesis, energy metabolism and bile production. The CFS patients could be subgrouped according to their lipid profiles (e.g., different profiles in those with acute onset compared with those with gradual onset). Some of the changes maybe due to viral reactivation or secondary infection.

The assessment of fatty acids and sterols in fasting plasma samples can indicate EFA deficits, suggest appropriate types of EFAs for supplementation, indicate potential cholesterol deficit associated anomalies, provide evidence for mitochondrial dysfunction and categorize CFS patients into biochemical subgroups. This can help to devise individually tailored management protocols.

Visual processing disability (scotopic vision) had been researched by Tim Roberts, Newcastle. The fact that patients with visual problems reported feeling better after taking antibiotics or amino acids led to a study investigating the possibility that biochemical anomalies in CFS correlated with visual processing anomalies. Urine excretion data revealed a number of biochemical abnormalities associated with symptom expression. These patients were shown to have Scotopic Sensitivity/Ihrlen Syndrome (SSIS) and it seems likely that there are specific biochemical markers. Hydroxyproline and proline were found to be significantly elevated. The lipid profiles also help in diagnosis and there was correlation with those suffering from conditions such as dyslexia and ADD with SSIS.

Children with reading difficulties (e.g., dyslexia) can be helped by the use of Ihrlen's filters. It is postulated that this approach maybe useful in CFS also, where there seems to be inadequate visual processing linked to dyslexia, with blurring and movement of print, and problems in the magno-cellular perceptual system. Use of colored lenses or cellophane or colored background to the computer screen, can have a major impact in improved reading ability and decrease in headaches. Different patients are found to need different colors. Amino acid supplementation and use of antioxidants may also be helpful. Pathogen elucidation and elimination can also be useful.

H. Kuratsune from Osaka, Japan and his team have studied acetyl-carnitine (ACC) levels for some time now, and have found that the majority of patients do have depleted serum levels. There is clear correlation between acetylcarnitine levels and rating score of fatigue in CFS. Acetylcarnitine is found (in mice) to be involved in the biosynthesis of major neurotransmitters like glutamate, aspartate and GABA. Acetylcarnitine metabolism and cerebral blood flow has been found to be deficient in Brodman's areas 9 and 24–areas of the brain associated with executive functions, such as affective and motivational behavior and attentive and autonomic functions.

RnaseL IN CFS

This session began with an overview by LeBleu (Montpellier, France) of the interferon-activated 2-5a/RnaseL pathway. Interierons have been characterised as mediators of a broad range of defence mechanisms particularly against viruses. Further evidence shows their involvement in immune regulation, cell growth and differentiation control.

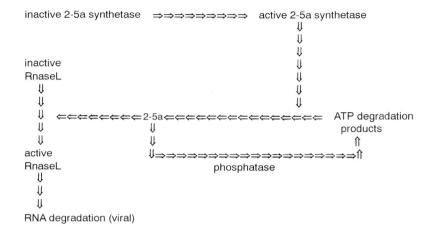

In CFS the RnaseL is a low molecular weight variety (normal is high molecular weight). The whole pathway is upregulated. RnaseL comprises 741 amino acids.

Robert Suhadolnik from Philadelphia continued to confirm his work that the RnaseL pathway is upregulated in CFS and has continued to demonstrate the presence of a low molecular weight (LMW) form of this enzyme in peripheral blood mononuclear cells (PBMC) in CFS. Two independent experimental methods were used to demonstrate the presence of this enzyme. Both methods demonstrated significantly statistical agreement with clinical diagnosis and showed a high degree of specificity and sensitivity. The levels of the LMW RnaseL correlated with Karnofsky scores. The presence of the LMW was independent of the duration of the CFS, and the CFS patients could be identified accurately. The drug Ampligen has been found to normalize the pattern.

K. De Meirleir also found the presence of LMW RnaseL in 680 of 705 patients studied. A more pronounced RnaseL dysfunction correlated with the 1988 definition for CFS–and this may relate to the more acute viral onset stressed in that definition. But RnaseL dysfunction also correlates significantly with those fulfilling the Fukuda definition. Presence of the abnormal enzyme also correlated with increased incidence of bronchial hyperactivity. Favorable outcome after ampligen treatment is inversely correlated with the presence of LMW RnaseL.

IMMUNOLOGY

The immunology session began with an overview of the immunological abnormalities in CFS by Nancy Klimas, Miami, USA.

There is always a trigger factor with 60-80% cases having acute onset with viral infection (e.g., EBV, CMV, Qfever, RRV, etc.). There maybe genetic predisposition. Psycho-neuro-immune mediators are important factors (e.g., stress preceding the illness is evident in 67% of patients).

The immune response is antigen driven and there is evidence of chronic immune activation, although the immune system is not wholly activated. Cytokines are the immune system's messengers and 3 types were described: cytotoxic/antiviral, promoters of antibody production and pro-inflammatory (which mediate inflammatory responses). The latter can affect sleep, which both the brain and immune systems require to function efficiently. There are changes in cytokine expression over time depending on illness severity. TNF-α receptor expression increases with flares of illness, and type 2 expression is increasingly evident as illness persists.

There are also indirect effects on the immune system such as soluble mediators, which act on many tissues, and influences from the brain and endocrine system. Long-term stress will lead to immune dysfunction, such as reduced CD8 cells, decreased NK function and changes in T cells. Depression also causes changes in immune function.

CFS is a model of neuro-endocrine-immune interaction with immune activation, autonomic changes and alterations in the HPA axis. The immune system is both a cause and effect interacting with the autonomic nervous system and the HPA axis. This suggests antigen exposure. Immune therapies, which shift the cytokine pattern to type 1 expression, should be considered.

Allergy in CFS was then discussed by J. Brostoff from London. Twenty-five percent of the population do suffer from intolerances/allergy and the percent is the same in CFS. He explained that food and inhalant sensitivity could lead to many health problems. Symptoms of intolerance include conditions such as migraine, irritable bowel, arthralgia and chronic fatigue. He recommended the value of trying elimination diets in helping establish whether or not a patient had intolerance. An interesting point was that diabetics rarely have allergies, and this may represent gene exclusion. He mentioned the effects of "exorphins" (external morphine-like substances) such as chocolate, which can have effects such as gut problems, addictive potential and psychological sequelae.

Multiple chemical sensitivity (MCS) which can be acute or lifelong was discussed. There is considerable overlap in symptoms with asthma, CFS, fibromyalgia, depression, somatisation disorder, hyperventilation syndrome. This presents problems with a case definition.

Hyperventilation syndrome occurs as a result of a patient with CFS being ill for a long time. There are many symptoms such as blurred vision, tachycardia, chest pain, pins and needles and yawning. He thinks the respiratory alkalosis leads to magnesium depletion, then muscle spasm. Noise sensitivity and vivid dreams often ensue.

Lambrecht from Ghent, Belgium, presented work on the clinical, immunological and neuro-imaging correlations in those with CFS. This was a very thorough investigation incorporating a wide range of medical and immunological investigations, Karnofsky performance ratings, pulmonary and exercises function, MRI and SPECT scanning. Physicians without knowledge of the clinical history evaluated the neuroSPECT scans. Two hundred ninety-four defects were found in 148 patients. Karnofsky scores correlated negatively with significant SPECT anomalies. Immune parameters were also positively correlated with scan results. Seventeen out of 30 patients had significant abnormalities on MR, with 10 times the number of lesions than in controls. The findings illustrate the multisystem involvement and disability in CFS supporting encephalomyelitic pathogenesis.

Byron Hyde (Canada) then discussed his findings in 16 CFS patients. He too found there were persisting major immunological abnormalities and a subgroup had associated abnormal brain SPECT scans. He then looked at the effects of the drug Isoprinosine on the immune markers in this subgroup. He found some of these patients had marked improvement in symptoms, with associated improvement in cytokine parameters and NK cell numbers. Improvement did not show in the placebo group.

Nickel allergy was discussed by B. Regland (Goteborg) as a possible marker for hyper-reactivity in women with CFS. Of those who reacted adversely to an antistaphylococcus vaccine used in treatment, 81% were found to be allergic to nickel (which was not present in the vaccine). Incidence of nickel allergy in healthy controls was 25%.

This was postulated as a possible area for further research. L. Sterz (Prague) looked at the presence of hypersensitivity to dental and environmental metals in those with CFS. He suggests that metal-driven inflammation may affect the HPA axis and indirectly symptoms characterizing chronic fatigue. Lymphocyte changes were shown in response to presence of mercury and nickel, and these improved in some patients when amalgam was removed. V. Stejskal (Stockholm) had also found significant numbers of metalspecific lymphocytes in the blood of patients with a CFS-like syndrome. This may be a genetic effect.

MICROBIOLOGY

Garth Nicolson (California) discussed diagnosis and treatment of cell-invasive mycoplasmal infections in CFS and related diseases. Consideration was given as to whether these infections are causative, cofactors or opportunistic. Mycoplasma penetrates right into the cells and plays havoc with the mitochondria. This leads to many symptoms. The most reliable and highly sensitive method of detection is by forensic PCR. Fifty percent of those suffering from Gulf War Illness (GWI) and family members with similar symptoms had evidence of mycoplasmal infections inside the Ieucocytes. In non-deployed healthy adults the incidence was 0-6%. *M. fermentans* was the most common species found.

Successful treatment of positive patients with long-term antibiotics was reviewed. Relapse was common in early cycles of treatment, but after up to seven 6-week cycles, those who were symptom free tested negative to mycoplasma. Sixty percent CFS/FM patients tested positive for mycoplasma compared to 6% of controls. Rheumatoid arthritic patients also tested 45% positive. It was concluded that treatment of these chronic conditions with antibiotics, oxidative therapy and nutritional supplements had potential for slow recovery. There were warnings about not using penicillin because of the increasing risk of reactions, including anaphylaxis.

Henry Butt (Newcastle) had investigated the changes in the distribution of anaerobic and aerobic bacteria, as well as the biochemical composition of faeces from patients with chronic fatigue and pain disorders. He found marked quantitative changes in both aerobic and anaerobic faecal microflora, with distributions significantly different to controls.

These alterations may adversely affect the symbiotic benefits that normally occur between microbes and host. Sixty percent CFS patients have gastrointestinal problems. The lipid composition of the stools in CFS showed significant correlation with gastrointestinal symptoms and changes in the distribution of gut flora. As a result, the clinician can evaluate gut dysfunction and devise individually tailored protocols.

It was interesting to note that less than 15% CFS patients had *Candida* in the faeces and none had evidence of overgrowth.

A further presentation on the effects of the coagulase negative staphylococcal membrane producing toxin by Hugh Dunstan (Newcastle, Australia) hypothesised that an occult pathogen maybe an aetiological agent contributing to the sustenance of fatigue and pain. Alterations in urine excretion and microbiology in CFS were investigated. Patients had multiple anomalies in amino and organic acid homeostasis, and it was possible to subgroup the CFS patients according to symptoms and characteristic urinary profile. The imbalances suggested active muscle catabolism, which was directly related to pain severity. The carriage of toxin producing coagulase negative staphylococci was strongly correlated to the catabolic response and pain severity.

Rickettsial infection had been found to have a possible link with CFS by C. Jadin (Johannensburg) following on the work of P. Bottero from Paris. There is similar clinical presentation between CFS, a number of auto-immune conditions and Rickettsial disease. When strains of rickettsia have been isolated, all patients in her clinic are treated with cyclical courses of antibiotics such as tetracyclines over several months. Good results are claimed.

W. A. Nix from Germany studied a group of 69 CFS patients who had proneness towards infections. Sixteen were found to have elevated titres for various viruses. In all patients a single-fibre electromyography (SFEMG) study was performed to ascertain whether there was a muscle membrane defect or neuromuscular transmission defect causing fatigue. SFEMG studies did not show abnormalities in either group of patients leading to the assumption that these defects are not likely to be the cause of the muscle fatigue in CFS.

DIAGNOSIS

Alterations in HPAaxis function were proposed by J. Gaab (Germany) as a shared pathway linking aetiological and perpetuating processes with observed physiological changes, such as immune function and central activation. Plasma cortisol, free cortisol and ACTH responses in response to stress and exercise were measured in CFS patients and controls. There was evidence for a lower "set-point" of HPA activity. There was no reduction in glucocorticoid secretion and no evidence for reduced glucocorticoid activity, and the changes in HPA activity are therefore likely to be central.

B. Hyde (Canada) reviewed the technological investigation of ME/CFS. He stressed the difficulties that many would have in accessing these tests. Twenty-five percent patients with acute onset tested positive by PCR for enteroviruses, while none did who had had gradual onset. Only 10% of his patients had a positive tilt table test. Red blood cell volume was reduced in 66% patients, meaning enormous implication for oxygen carriage. Blood volume was reduced on average to 60% of normal. He confirmed that immunological tests are expensive and difficult.

Tim Roberts and the Newcastle, NSW team had investigated erythrocyte oxidative damage in CFS. These patients had increased levels of methaemoglobin and malondiahyde as markers of oxidative stress and had increased mean erythrocyte volume compared to controls. Erythrocyte distribution risk was a primary factor differentiating controls and sub-groups of those with CFS. These parameters were associated with symptom expression and symptom indices in the patients. The data suggest that oxidative stress maybe a contributor in the pathology of a subset of CFS patients. This may indicate persistent underlying intracellular infection. Antioxidant therapy maybe therefore be useful in some CFS patients.

Pituitary function was studied by G. Moorkens and his team (Antwerp). Comprehensive hormone testing was performed in 73 patients with 21 controls. Significant changes in growth hormone (GH) secretion were demonstrated during insulin tolerance testing and nocturnal GH secretion. Increase in visceral fat (measured by CT scan), a characteristic of GH deficiency, was clearly demonstrated. It is possible that this decrease in GH in CFS is related to poor sleep.

CLINICAL OBSERVATIONS

S. Bastien (California) tested for motor abnormalities associated with neuropsychologically compromised CFS patients. She used an extensive neuropsychological battery, and found most motor tests were impaired bilaterally. On the majority of motor indicators, the dominant hand performance was worse than the non-dominant. Male results were slightly different to the females. The results support the patient complaints of clumsiness, dropping things, weakness and slowed motor coordination.

Fluctuations in fatigue were described as a result of a French fatigue questionnaire by J. Cabane (Paris). Among the 10 patients, none had permanent fatigue and all had more than one period of fatigue per 24 hours. Various rhythms of fatigue were noted such as monthly, weekly and daily.

Memory impairment was examined by John de Luca (New Jersey) to see whether there is deficient learning of information in CFS as opposed to deficit in retrieval from long-term storage. A well controlled study was described. The results implied that the primary problem in CFS results from deficient acquisition as the patients required significantly more trials to learn a word list than did healthy controls, but there was also some deficient retrieval from long-term storage.

J. Hardt (Mainz, Germany) reported on the work undertaken in 3 countries to compare the quality of life of CFS patients. Remarkable similarity in self-rated functional status suggests homogeneity in CFS patients in USA, Germany and UK.

Byron Hyde (Canada) reported on 4 patients who fell ill with CFS and 4 who fell ill with MS immediately after recombinant Hepatitis B immunisation. The onset in the 8 patients was identical, but the CFS group were distinguishable, as SPECT scan changes were evident with normal MRIs, while demyelinating lesions were evident in the MS patients. The question was raised as to whether the effects after immunisation were coincidental or causal. As a result of similar worries in France this type of vaccine for children has been withdrawn. However it was pointed out that we should not forget the enormous and important benefits in preventative immunisation programmes.

Altered perception of muscle force in patients with CFS was discussed by W. Nix (Germany). CFS patients perceived that it was more difficult to generate a given force output than normals, and although the recovery phase was slower in the CFS patients, they could in fact perform as well as the controls. Its seems therefore that the fatigue could be perceptual and the possibility was raised that mental fatigue sets in earlier than the physical fatigue.

A significant degree of functional impairment was demonstrated in CFS patients surveyed by N. Posner and his team in Queensland. They used the SF36 and found particularly that these patients had significant physical role limitation. Eight dimensions were assessed and the means for each were markedly lower than the population norms. The least differences were in the mental health and emotional role limitation dimensions. Results were dissimilar from most other disease profiles, particularly depression, and indicate a very significant degree of functional impairment. Support needs should thus be recognized.

K. Rowe (Melbourne) looked at whether the symptom complex of adult CFS occurs in adolescents. She studied 189 young people with defined onset of fatigue with a symptom complex lasting at least 6 months. Eighty-five of patients had an illness following an acute viral illness. Factor analysis was used with the data from the clinical group. Symptoms reported were consistent across all subjects, and while the symptoms in CFS were similar to adults, prolonged fatigue after exercise, headache, concentration difficulties, disturbed sleep, abdominal pain and myalgia were particularly evident. Somatization disorder was not a likely alternative because of low response frequencies of such symptoms.

Two papers on exercise capacity in CFS were then presented. P. deBecker (Brussels) et al. found that CFS patients were limited in their capacity to perform physical activities. Females were on average more impaired than males. Exercise parameters were generally down with a mean working capacity of approximately 55% of normal. C. Sargent (Adelaide, SA) found that CFS patients were not deconditioned and a graded exercise training programme would seem unwarranted in treatment. These patients had normal exercise capacity with abnormal lactic acid accumulation demonstrated from the beginning of the exercise.

TREATMENT

Treatment of rickettsial and chlamydial infections with macrolides and/or cyclines was discussed by P. Bottero (Paris). Symptoms may be accentuated initially due to release of bacterial toxins, but this can be combatted by the use of antiinflammatory drugs. The drugs are used cyclically and may be needed for one to two years to obtain positive outcome. Overall results were not discussed.

Treatment with the drug Isoprinosine (an immune modulator with anti-viral properties) was outlined by B. Hyde (Canada), who described this drug as having been available for 30 years without encountering any serious side effects. Patients studied were widely and thoroughly investigated, and a group of 16 CFS patients with abnormal SPECT scans was treated using placebo control over a 7 month period. Seven patients improved on the drug, 7 remained unchanged and 2 deteriorated when on placebo, with improvement once the drug was reinstated. Improvements in general health and energy were modest but significant. All those who improved were happy to continue. Thinking and memory improved, ataxia decreased, headaches decreased, there was less clumsiness and better motor function. In particular, ability to attend social functions increased. Only one patient experienced side effects, which were bad headaches.

N. Klimas (Miami) discussed further her work showing alteration of type1/type2 cytokine patterns following adoptive immunotherapy using expanded lymph node cells. Thirteen patients with strict inclusion criteria were studied. Lymph nodes were removed and cells were then cultured for 10-12 days and reinfused into the donor who was monitored for safety and possible clinical benefit. No adverse events were recorded. Two patients had unsuitable fibrotic lymph nodes, so were not included. For the remaining 11 who underwent successful expansion and reinfusion, there were favourable clinical and immunological results. It is hoped that further trials will follow.

Three studies regarding the use of the drug Ampligen were then reported. Ampligen is a biological response modifier with antiviral and immunomodulatory effects. D. Strayer (USA) had compared twice or thrice weekly infusions in order to optimize the dosing schedule. One hundred and eleven patients were studied. Activity and safety of the 2 dosing schedules were compared and it was found that thrice weekly dosing offers no advantage over a twice weekly schedule. There were slightly more adverse events in the thrice weekly group, mainly myalgia and flu-like symptoms. A pharmaco-economic analysis intervention in CFS was presented by W. Carter (USA) looking at the savings on concommitant medications and hospitalisation in the treated and untreated groups. Although the cost of the drug is extremely high, considerable savings were shown to be made in these areas, which it seems could have some thrust in convincing government agencies of the potential of this drug, particularly more so if patients could eventually return to the workforce.

Finally, K. De Meirleir presented his work on the Ampligen study in Belgium. Forty-four severely affected patients under 60 had been given the drug for 24 weeks and compared to 16 untreated controls. Infusions were given twice weekly starting with 200 mg and increasing to 400 mg. There was significant improvement in bicycle-exercise testing, increased Karnofsky scores, reduction in cognitive impairment, alleviation of many of the CFS symptoms and improved general health perception, significant improvement in day to day function and no serious adverse events.

POSTERS

A wide variety of posters were displayed and the following represents a brief overview of some of the important findings.

Epidemiology

P. de Becker (Brussels) looked at mode of disease onset in CFS. Seventy-four percent patients had acute onset with progressive disease in 26%. Infectious agents seem to play an important role in the onset of CFS with other factors such as immune dysregulation involved in the perpetuation of the illness. He also did a 6 month follow up in CFS patients. He found that health stayed unchanged or deteriorated measured by several parameters. Especially, physical capacity seemed to get worse over time. Only a small number of patients were followed over this relatively short period of time. One thousand two hundred and forty-eight patients were studied in a further poster by de Becker, and in almost all patients all symptoms of the Holmes criteria occurred. Other symptoms noted were: dyspnoea, lightheadedness, gastro-intestinal complaints, cold extremities, decreased libido and disequalibrium. They found the Fukuda definition less stringent and therefore less suitable for scientific homogeneity.

E. Fitzgibbon (Galway, Ireland) had used the SF36 in a postal survey of 123 CFS patients. There was 77% response rate. With a mean duration of illness of 5 years, 66% were improving, 29% were static and the remainder were worse. Twenty-six percent described themselves as almost back to normal with 60% back to fulltime work or study. The females had worse general health and reported more symptoms. Quality of life was lower in all domains measured by the

SF36 than norms, and the overall results were unique compared to data from other disease groups.

In the UK the diagnosis of CFS seems better accepted than Multiple Chemical Sensitivity as pointed out by D. Jones. Seventy-eight patients had completed questionnaires demonstrating the difficulties in diagnosis and the complexity of this condition. Many possible causes were cited. She had also followed up 45 patients who attributed their CFS-like illness to use of cotrimoxazole.

Midlife and elderly women's vulnerability to CFS was discussed by M. van Moffaert (Ghent, Belgium). It seems many underlying health disorders and sociological factors increase the vulnerability to both CFS and multisomatoform disorders.

Immunology

Prevalence of bronchial hyper-responsiveness in CFS was observed by K. Bervoets (Brussels). A high incidence was observed irrespective of smoking habits. This finding cannot be explained by the expiratory muscle effort involved in the histamine provocation procedure, as there was no significant difference between baseline spirometry and expiratory muscle strength between CFS patients and controls. E. Brouns furthered this work by looking to see if there was correlation between cellular immunity and bronchial hyper-reactivity in CFS. These patients were significantly found to have an increased number of activated T-cells and a decreased number of cytotoxic T-cells.

RnaseL testing was done in 136 German patients by L. Habets. RnaseL dysfunction was found in most patients with a correlation between the RnaseL/LMW RnaseL ratio and disease symptoms. M. Reynders (Brussels) found that the large amount of LMW RnaseL correlates with higher levels of IFN gamma, which has antiviral properties. Normal NK cell numbers with high LMW/HMW ratio correlate with high IL-12 levels in CFS patients compared with controls. IL-12 has been shown to be a potent inducer of IFN gamma secretion by both resting and activated T and NK cells in humans.

Biochemistry

D. Racciati (Italy) et al. observed an alteration in the antioxidative enzyme activities of skeletal muscle, and alterations of fatty acid composition and fluidity of membrane in muscles in CFS and FM patients.

No similar abnormalities were found in controls. The oxidative muscle damage could represent the consequence of an impaired oxidative/antioxidative system and could possible correlate with the increased muscle fatiguability in CFS.

Endocrinology

Four case reports by A. D. Hock (Germany) brought up the possibility that Vitamin D and parathormone disturbance should not be overlooked as a possible cause of chronic fatigue. The symptoms are very similar and this is a treatable disorder.

S. Meghan (Boston) as leader of a group of female health care workers with CFS stressed the importance of considering that as this illness seemed to be "predominantly female" we should not overlook the impact of the endocrine system as a likely factor in potentiating CFS.

Clinical Observations

Symptom patterns in adolescents with CFS were again addressed by K. Rowe (Melbourne). One hundred and eighty-nine young people were studied. Three subgroups were identified according to severity. The more severe group had greater fatigue and pain, the moderately severe group having more neurocognitive symptoms and the least severe having more headaches, nausea and abdominal pain. Investigation of these subgroups may assist with management.

The pregnancy experiences of women with CFS were explored by R. Vallings (Auckland, NZ). Most women found the experiences positive, but the importance of family and partner support was emphasised together with an understanding of CFS by the obstetric personnel involved.

Data were collected by P. de Becker and de Meirleir (Brussels) on 1248 patients attending a clinic complaining of chronic fatigue. The patients were subgrouped after thorough review according to whether they had CFS or chronic fatigue from other disease causes. Frequency and severity of symptoms were more marked in the CFS group. The physical capacity of the CFS patients was lower and they seemed to be more debilitated. In another paper they also found that 4.5% of a large cohort of patients reported that their illness came on following surgery with an accompanying transfusion. None had developed Hepatitis C or other possible transfusion-transmitted infection. The findings do point to a possible transmissable cause in this subset of CFS patients. They therefore advise CFS patients not to offer to be blood donors. Blood transfusions also should be given when strictly necessary. While looking at possible opportunistic infections, they concluded that mycoplasmas might be partially responsible for some of the signs and symptoms in CFS. They also seem to be implicated in the T-cell activation observed in these patients.

CFS patients suffer significantly from psychomotor dysfunction, which may contribute to the global disability in the syndrome (L. Lambrecht, Ghent). Rehabilitation methods including biofeedback and progressive aerobic training and restoring psychomotor abilities may constitute an important part of management. Low prevalence of autonomic dysfunction was found in this group of patients. The same team had evaluated neuropsychological impairment using numerous different tests and found that the Purdue pegboard turned out to be the most affected test. Visual memory span was affected and 20% of the patients were depressed according to the Beck depression inventory. When they reviewed SPECTscans in CFS patients, 189 aberrations were found in 65 patients.

O. Zachrisson (Sweden) found a high prevalence of irritable bowel syndrome in CFS and FM patients (61%) and a further 19% had other GI symptoms. A common pathogenic mechanism such as disturbed microflora in the gut was suggested.

Management

L. Barker (Essex, UK) described an 8 week group programme for CFS patients was followed up by questionnaire/audit, and results demonstrated that 71% patients improved, with a number returning to work or college. It is hoped therefore to develop outpatient services to provide a comprehensive management approach to the illness.

P. Bottero (Paris) demonstrated the immunology of Rickettsial diseases (small intracellular gram-negative bacteria). It seems that rickettsiae penetrate and persist in the macrophages and diminish their function. Accompanying immunological changes also occur.

GULF WAR SYNDROME

Four papers on Gulf War Illness (GWI) were presented as part of the opening symposium.

Peckerman and Natelson (Orange, USA) presented figures to familiarise us with the situation in the USA. Almost seventeen percent of returning veterans surveyed had medical problems. The rate of Chronic Fatigue in this group was 5.2% compared to 1.2% of veterans in non-active service. Of those diagnosed as suffering from GWI 50% fitted the criteria for a diagnosis of CFS. It was hypothesised that those suffering from GWI have poor control of cardiovascular stress. Cardiovascular regulation was studied using various approaches. BP tended to fall during speech and mental arithmetic tests with no difference in pressor tests. During the speech test the peripheral resistance did not budge as it should. Three possible issues were raised: Is this: (1) related to the cause of fatigue, (2) a marker of illness or (3) a premorbid condition? The greatest physiological consequences, impacting central and peripheral control systems, occurred in veterans who sustained exposure to both chemical and severe psychological war stresses.

Using factor analysis, Paul Levene (Washington) also concluded that the identification of a cluster of neurologic symptoms in a large sample (7000) of deployed Gulf War vets that could not be found in non-deployed vets supports the possibility that environmental factors could be responsible for some of the complaints of Gulf War veterans.

M. Hooper (UK) described the Gulf War as the most toxic war in all military history. Up to 17 vaccines were given, many disinfectants were used (e.g., in insect control), many chemical warfare agents were in the area, "uranium," weapons were used creating toxic dust, biological weaponry was in the area (e.g., brucella, smallpox, viruses) and many other chemical agents (smoke, oilfires) were prevalent. Birth defects have now been found to be a major factor in Iraqi veterans' families. Risks of leukaemia, other cancers, neurotoxic effects and possible effects on sperm are also becoming evident.

G. Nicolson pointed out that there is as yet no case definition for GWI, but the signs and symptoms loosely fit the CFS definition. Using Forensic PCR Hybridization it was found that 45% GWI patients showed evidence of mycoplasmal infections in the leucocytes but not in the plasma or serum. When comparing CFS patients, 70% of them were found positive for mycoplasma. A variety of mycoplasma species were found. These infections could be causative, cofactors or opportunistic. These infections maybe a major source of morbidity in these related illnesses. There is some evidence of possible transmission to family members. Possible other transmittable bacterial and viral infections maybe involved.

Treatment with appropriate antibiotics and nutritional support can result in improvement in these chronic conditions, though not in every case. It is possible that GWI is to a large degree due to multiple exposure to chemical, radiological and biological agents that can cause immune depression, multiple infections, and multifactorial illnesses, which maybe treatable.

Role of Mycoplasmal Infections
in Fatigue Illnesses:
Chronic Fatigue and Fibromyalgia
Syndromes, Gulf War Illness
and Rheumatoid Arthritis

G. L. Nicolson, PhD
M. Y. Nasralla, PhD
A. R. Franco, MD
K. De Meirleir, MD, PhD
N. L. Nicolson, PhD
R. Ngwenya, MD
J. Haier, MD, PhD

G. L. Nicolson and M. Y. Nasralla are affiliated with The Institute for Molecular Medicine, Huntington Beach, CA 92649 USA.

A. R. Franco is affiliated with the Arthritis Center of Riverside, Riverside, CA 92501 USA.

K. De Meirleir is affiliated with the Internal Medicine, Free University of Brussels, 1090 Brussels, Belgium.

N. L. Nicolson is affiliated with The Institute for Molecular Medicine, Huntington Beach, CA 92649 USA.

R. Ngwenya is affiliated with the James Mobb Immune Enhancement, Harare, Zimbabwe.

J. Haier is affiliated with The Institute for Molecular Medicine, Huntington Beach, CA 92649 USA.

Address correspondence to: Prof. G. L. Nicolson, The Institute for Molecular Medicine, 15162 Triton Lane, Huntington Beach, CA 92649 (E-mail: gnicimm@ix.netcom.com).

[Haworth co-indexing entry note]: "Role of Mycoplasmal Infections in Fatigue Illnesses: Chronic Fatigue and Fibromyalgia Syndromes, Gulf War Illness and Rheumatoid Arthritis." Nicolson, G. L. et al. Co-published simultaneously in *Journal of Chronic Fatigue Syndrome* (The Haworth Medical Press, an imprint of The Haworth Press, Inc.) Vol. 6, No. 3/4, 2000, pp. 23-39; and: *Chronic Fatigue Syndrome: Critical Reviews and Clinical Advances* (ed: Kenny De Meirleir, and Roberto Patarca-Montero) The Haworth Medical Press, an imprint of The Haworth Press, Inc., 2000, pp. 23-39. Single or multiple copies of this article are available for a fee from The Haworth Document Delivery Service [1-800-342-9678, 9:00 a.m. - 5:00 p.m. (EST). E-mail address: getinfo@haworthpressinc.com].

SUMMARY. Bacterial and viral infections are purported to be associated with several fatigue illnesses, including Chronic Fatigue Syndrome (CFS), Fibromyalgia Syndrome (FMS), Gulf War Illnesses (GWI) and Rheumatoid Arthritis (RA), as causative agents, cofactors or opportunistic infections. We and others have looked for the presence of invasive pathogenic mycoplasmal infections in patients with CFS, FMS, GWI and RA and have found significantly more mycoplasmal infections in CFS, FMS, GWI and RA patients than in healthy controls. Most patients had multiple mycoplasmal infections (more than one species). Patients with chronic fatigue as a major sign often have different clinical diagnoses but display overlapping signs/symptoms similar to many of those found in CFS/FMS. When a chronic fatigue illness, such as GWI, spreads to immediate family members, they present with similar signs/symptoms and mycoplasmal infections. CFS/FMS/GWI patients with mycoplasmal infections generally respond to particular antibiotics (doxycycline, minocycline, ciprofloxacin, azithromycin and clarithromycin), and their long-term administration plus nutritional support, immune enhancement and other supplements appear to be necessary for recovery. Examination of the efficacy of antibiotics in recovery of chronic illness patients reveals that the majority of mycoplasma-positive patients respond and many eventually recover. Other chronic infections, such as viral infections, may also be involved in various chronic fatigue illnesses with or without mycoplasmal and other bacterial infections, and these multiple infections could be important in causing patient morbidity and difficulties in treating these illnesses. *[Article copies available for a fee from The Haworth Document Delivery Service: 1-800-342-9678. E-mail address: <getinfo@haworthpressinc.com> Website: <http://www.haworthpressinc.com>]*

KEYWORDS. Mycoplasma, Gulf War syndrome, fibromyalgia, rheumatoid arthritis, antibiotics

INTRODUCTION

Many debilitating chronic illnesses are characterized by the presence of chronic fatigue (1). Indeed, chronic fatigue is the most commonly reported medical complaint of all patients seeking medical care (2). However, the fatigue syndromes, such as Chronic Fatigue Syndrome (CFS, sometimes called Myalgic Encephalomyelitis), Fibromyalgia Syndrome (FMS) and Gulf War Illnesses (GWI) are distinguishable as separate syndromes that have muscle and overall fatigue as major characteristics, among many other multiorgan signs and symptoms (3-6), including immune system abnormalities (7). These syndromes have complex chronic signs and symptoms, including muscle pain, chronic fatigue, headaches, memory loss, nausea, gastrointestinal problems, joint pain, vision problems, breathing problems, depression, low grade fevers, skin disorders, tissue swelling, chemical sensitivities, among others. Because of the complex nature of these illnesses, many patients are often diagnosed with multiple syndromes. Unfortunately, due to the lack of definitive laboratory or clinical tests that could identify the cause(s) of these illnesses, many patients are diagnosed with somatoforensic disorders. Often these patients have cognitive problems, such as short term memory loss, difficulty concentrating and psychological problems, that in the absence of contrary laboratory tests can result in practitioners diagnosing somatoform disorders rather than organic problems (6). Stress is often portrayed as an important factor in these disorders, and in fact stress can have many effects on the hormonal and immune systems that could be detrimental in virtually any chronic illness (8).

There is growing awareness that the chronic fatigue illnesses can have an infectious nature that is either responsible (causative) for the illness, a cofactor for the illness or appears as an opportunistic infection(s) responsible for aggravating patient morbidity (9). There are several reasons for this notion (10), including the nonrandom or clustered appearance of the illness, often in immediate family members, and the course of the illness and its response to therapies based on treatment of infectious agents. Since chronic illnesses are often complex, involving multiple, nonspecific, overlapping signs and symptoms, they are difficult to diagnose and even more difficult to treat (9). Most chronic fatigue illnesses do not have effective therapies, and these patients rarely recover from their condition (11), causing in some cases catastrophic economic problems.

SIGNS AND SYMPTOMS ANALYSIS

Some chronic illnesses, such as Rheumatoid Arthritis (RA), are well established in their clinical profile (12), whereas others, such as CFS, FMS and GWI, have rather nonspecific but similar overlapping, multi-organ signs and symptoms. A major difference between these illnesses appears to be in the severity of specific signs and symptoms. For example, CFS patients most often complain of chronic fatigue and joint pain, stiffness and soreness, whereas FMS patients have as their major complaint muscle and overall pain, soreness and weakness. For the most part, the clinical profiles of these illnesses are similar, and this can be easily seen when the signs and symptoms of CFS, FMS, and GWI patients are compared (Figures 1A and 1B). Thus, although chronic illnesses are considered to be complex, they do display certain similarities, suggesting that these illnesses are related and not completely separate syndromes (6,9). In addition, these chronic illness patients often show increased sensitivities to various environmental irritants and chemicals and enhanced allergic responses.

Although chronic fatigue illnesses have been known in the literature for many years, most patients with CFS, FMS, GWI and in some cases RA have had few treatment options. This may have been due to the imprecise nature of their diagnoses, which are usually based primarily on clinical observations rather than laboratory tests, and a lack of understanding about the underlying causes of these illnesses or the factors responsible for patient morbidity. Chronic illnesses could have different initial causes or triggers but similar secondary events, such as opportunistic viral and/or bacterial infections that cause significant morbidity (9,10). With time, these secondary events may progress to be the most important in determining overall signs and symptoms and treatment options.

The data presented in Figures 1A and 1B show the most common signs and symptoms found in CFS, FMS and GWI patients and symptomatic GWI family members after the onset of illness. In these figures the data for FMS and CFS have been combined, because previous studies indicated that with the exception of the extent of muscle pain and tenderness, there were essentially no major differences in patient signs (6,10). Illness Survey Forms were analyzed to determine the most common signs and symptoms at the time when blood was drawn from patients. The intensity of approximately 120 patient signs and symptoms prior to and after onset of illness was recorded on a 10-point rank scale (0-10, extreme). The data were arranged into 29 different signs and symptoms groups and were considered positive if the average value after onset of illness was two or more points higher than prior to the onset of illness. CFS/FMS patients had complex signs and symptoms that were similar to those reported for GWI, and the presence of rheumatoid signs and symptoms in each of these disorders indicates that there are also similarities to RA (12,13). Moreover, it is not unusual to find immediate family members who slowly displayed

FIGURE 1A. Incidence of increase in severity of signs and symptoms in 260 chronic illness patients. Severity of illness was scored using 117 signs and symptoms on a 10-point scale (0, none; 10 extreme) prior to and after the onset of illness. Scores were placed into 29 categories containing 3-9 signs/symptoms and were recorded as the sum of differences between values before and after onset of illness divided by the number of questions in the category. Changes in score values of 2 or more points were considered relevant. Patient groups were CFS/FMS (■), GWI (▨), GWI symptomatic family members (▩), and chronic illness patients not in the above groups that did not show evidence of chronic bacterial infection (□). Asterisk (*) indicates score = 0.

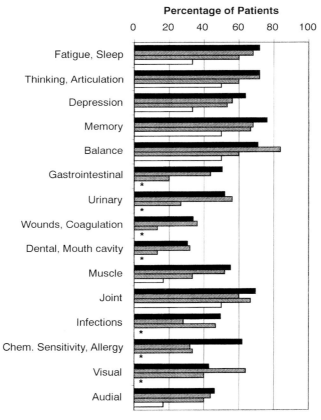

Increase in Signs and Symtpoms I

FIGURE 1B. Incidence of increase in severity of signs and symptoms in 260 chronic illness patients. Severity of illness was scored using 117 signs and symptoms on a 10-point scale (0, none; 10 extreme) prior to and after the onset of illness. Scores were placed into 29 categories containing 3-9 signs/symptoms and were recorded as the sum of differences between values before and after onset of illness divided by the number of questions in the category. Changes in score values of 2 or more points were considered relevant. Patient groups were CFS/FMS (■), GWI (▨), GWI symptomatic family members (▧), and chronic illness patients not in the above groups that did not show evidence of chronic bacterial infection (□). Asterisk (*) indicates score = 0.

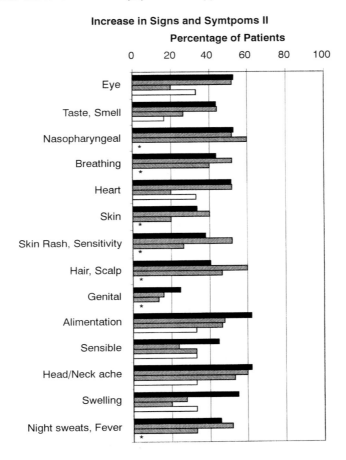

similar signs and symptoms following the return home of veterans with GWI, suggesting that these civilian patients contracted their illnesses from chronically ill family members with GWI (10). Examination of the increase in signs and symptoms of GWI family members that now have a chronic illness similar to GWI indicates that they have signs and symptoms similar to civilian CFS/FMS patients. The main difference between veterans with GWI and their family members was in the greater breadth and severity of signs and symptoms found in GWI patients than in their symptomatic family members. Since Gulf War veterans were presumably exposed to many more environmental toxic agents compared to nondeployed family members, this is not unexpected. When the signs and symptoms of CFS/FMS/GWI were compared to patients with other chronic illnesses that did not show evidence of chronic infections, there were also notable differences. For example, in contrast to CFS/FMS/GWI patients, this latter chronic illness patient group did not show differences in gastrointestinal problems, coagulation problems, hair loss and scalp problems, night sweats and intermittent fevers (Figures 1A and 1B). This suggests that CFS/FMS/GWI patients with chronic infections may have some unique clinical problems not commonly found in other chronic illness patients.

CHRONIC INFECTIONS IN CFS, FMS AND GWI

As stated above, there exists indirect evidence suggesting the infectious nature in at least certain subsets of chronic illness patients. We have been particularly interested in the association of specific chronic infectious agents with CFS, FMS, GWI and RA, because these microorganisms can potentially cause most or essentially all of the signs and symptoms found in these patients (6,9,10,13). One type of "stealth" infection that could fulfill the criteria of association with a wide range of signs and symptoms are certain microorganisms of the class Mollicutes. This is a class of small bacteria, lacking cell walls, and some species are capable of invading several types of human cells and tissues and are associated with a wide variety of human diseases (14).

We and others have examined the presence of mycoplasmal blood infections in CFS, FMS, GWI and RA patients. The clinical diagnosis of these disorders was obtained from referring physicians according to the patients' major signs and symptoms. Blood was collected, shipped over night at $4\,^{\circ}$C and processed immediately for Nucleoprotein Gene Tracking (NPGT) after isolation of blood leukocyte nuclei (15,16) or Forensic Polymerase Chain Reaction (FPCR) after purification of blood leukocyte DNA using a Chelex procedure (6,13,17). We used FPCR to determine the species of mycoplasmal infections. The sensitivity and specificity of the PCR methods were determined by examining serial dilutions of purified DNA of *M. fermentans, M. pneumoniae, M. penetrans* and *M. hominis.* Amounts as low as 10 fg of purified DNA were detectable. The amplification with genus primers produced the expected fragment size in all tested species, which was confirmed by hybridization with an inner probe (18). Others have also used PCR with single (19,20) or multiple (21,22) sets of PCR primers. Using NPGT to analyze the blood leukocytes from GWI patients we found that 91/200 (~ 45%) were positive for mycoplasmal infections. In contrast, in non-deployed, healthy adults the incidence of mycoplasmal infections was 4/62 (~ 6%) (15,16) (Table 1). Similarly, using PCR 55% of GWI patients were positive for *Mycoplasma* spp. and 36% were found to have *M. fermentans* infections (22) (Table 1). The slight difference in percentage of positive patients is probably due to the differences in sensitivities of these two methods. In comparison, using FPCR or PCR 52-63% of CFS/FMS patients (n~1,000) had mycoplasmal infections (6,19-23), whereas only 9-15% of controls (n~450) tested positive (Table 1).

Patients with CFS/FMS often have multiple mycoplasmal infections and probably other chronic infections as well. When we examined CFS/FMS patients for the presence of *M. fermentans, M. pneumoniae, M. penetrans, M. hominis* infections, multiple infections were found in over one-half of 93 patients (17) (Table 1). CFS/FMS patients had double (> 30%) or triple (> 20%) mycoplasmal infections, but only when one of the species was *M. fermentans* or *M. pneumoniae* (17). We also found higher score values for increases in the severity of signs and symptoms in CFS/FMS patients with multiple infections. CFS/FMS patients with multiple mycoplasmal infections generally had a longer history of illness, suggesting that patients may have contracted additional infections during their illness (17).

CHRONIC INFECTIONS IN RA

The causes of rheumatoid diseases are not known, but RA and other autoimmune diseases could be triggered or more likely exacerbated by

TABLE 1. Summary of mycoplasmal infections in patient groups and controls.

Percentage of Subjects Positive for Mycoplasmal Infections

Reference / Method	(A) NPGT	(B) NPGT	(C) FPCR	(D) FPCR	(E) FPCR	(F) PCR	(G) PCR	(H) PCR	(I) PCR	(J) FPCR
Gulf War Illness (n)	(30)	(170)							(60)	
M. spp.	47	45							55	
M. fermentans	31	30							36	
M. pneumoniae										
M. hominis									5	
M. penetrans									3	
CFS/FMS (n)			(132)	(91)*		(200)	(50)	(100)	(140)	(565)
M. spp.			63	100*			54	54	52-54	53
M. fermentans			50	48*		67	36	36	32-35	25
M. pneumoniae				59*						
M. hominis				31*					8-9	
M. penetrans				19*					4-6	
Rheumatoid Arthritis (n)					(28)				(60)	
M. spp.									49	
M. fermentans					53				23	
M. pneumoniae					29					
M. hominis					18				11	
M. penetrans					21				7	
					4					
Controls (n)	(14)	(41)	(32)	(33)	(32)	(77)	(50)	(100)	(160)	(71)
M. spp.	0	4.8	9			16.8	14	15	15	9.9
M. fermentans	0		9	9	9		8	8	8	2.8
M. pneumoniae			0	0	0					
M. hominis				0	0			3	3	
M. penetrans				0	0			2	2	
				0	0					

Method: NPGT, Nucleoprotein Gene Tracking; FPCR, Forensic Polymerase Chain Reaction; PCR, Polymerase Chain Reaction. **References:** A, Nicolson and Nicolson, 1996 (15); B, Nicolson et al., 1998 (16); C, Nicolson et al., 1998 (6); D, Nasralla et al., 1999 (17); E, Haier et al., 1999 (13); F, Huang et al., 1999 (20); G, Vojdani et al., 1998 (19); H, Choppa et al., 1998 (21); I, Vojdani and Franco, 1999 (22); J, Nasralla et al., 1999 (23). *Only patients that were positive for *Mycoplasma* spp. were enrolled in the study.

infectious agents (24). In some animal species infection by certain species of mycoplasmas can result in remarkable clinical and pathological similarities to RA and other rheumatic diseases. Aerobic and anaerobic intestinal bacteria, viruses and mycoplasmas have been proposed as important agents in RA (24-29), and there has been increasing evidence that mycoplasmas may play a role in the initiation or progression of RA (13,29-31). Mycoplasmas have been proposed to interact non-specifically with B-lymphocytes, resulting in modulation of immunity, autoimmune reactions and promotion of rheumatic diseases (30), and mycoplasmas have been found in the joint tissues of patients with rheumatic diseases, suggesting their pathogenic involvement (28).

When Haier et al. (13) and Vojdani and Franco (22) examined RA patients' blood leukocytes for the presence of mycoplasmas, it was found that approximately one-half were infected with various species of mycoplasmas. The most common species found was *M. fermentans*, followed by *M. pneumoniae* and *M. hominis* and finally *M. penetrans* (13,22). Similar to what we reported in CFS/FMS patients (17), there was a high percentage of multiple mycoplasmal infections in RA patients when one of the species was *M. fermentans* (13).

The precise role of mycoplasmas in RA and other rheumatic inflammatory diseases is under investigation; however, mycoplasmas could be important cofactors in the development of inflammatory responses in rheumatic diseases and for progression of RA. As an example of the possible role of mycoplasmas in rheumatic diseases, *M. arthritidis* infections in animals can trigger and exacerbate autoimmune arthritis (31,32). This mycoplasma can also suppress T-cells and release substances that act on polymorphonuclear granulocytes, such as oxygen radicals, chemotactic factors and other substances (32). Mycoplasmal infections can increase proinflammatory cytokines, such as Interleukin-1, -2 and -6 (33), suggesting that they are involved in the development and possibly progression of rheumatic diseases such as RA.

A variety of microorganisms have been under investigation as cofactors or causative agents in rheumatic diseases (9,24,25). The discovery of EB virus (26) and cytomegalovirus (27) in the cells of the synovial lining in RA patients suggested their involvement in RA, possibly as a cofactor. There are a number of bacteria and viruses that are candidates in the induction or progression of RA (9,24). In support of a bacterial involvement in RA, antibiotics like minocycline can alleviate the clinical signs and symptoms of RA (34). This and similar drugs are likely suppressing infections of sensitive microorganisms like mycoplasmas in rheumatic diseases, although they could also have other (anti-inflammatory and immunomodulatory) effects.

MYCOPLASMAL INFECTIONS IN OTHER DISEASES

Mycoplasmas have been associated with the progression of autoimmune and immunosuppressive diseases, such as HIV-AIDS (35). In some cases these infections have been associated with terminal human diseases, such as an acute fatal illness found with *M. fermentans* infections in non-AIDS patients (36). Importantly, mycoplasmal infections are now thought to be a major source of morbidity in HIV-AIDS (37). On this basis, Blanchard and Montagnier (37) have proposed that certain mycoplasmas like *M. fermentans* are important cofactors in the progression of HIV-AIDS, accelerating disease progression and accounting, in part, for the increased susceptibility of AIDS patients to additional opportunistic infections. Since most studies on the incidence of mycoplasmal infections in HIV-AIDS patients have employed relatively insensitive tests, it is likely that the occurrence of mycoplasmal infections in HIV-AIDS is much greater than previously thought and may be associated with a rapid fatal course of the disease. In HIV-AIDS, mycoplasmas like *M. fermentans* can cause renal and CNS complications (38), and mycoplasmas have been found in various tissues, such as the respiratory epithelial cells of AIDS patients (39). Other species of mycoplasmas have been found in AIDS patients where they have also been associated with disease progression (40). In addition to immune suppression, some of this increased pathogenecity may be the result of mycoplasma-induced host cell membrane damage from toxic oxygenated products released from intracellular mycoplasmas (41). Also, mycoplasmas may regulate the HIV-1 virus, such as HIV-LTR-dependent gene expression (42), suggesting that mycoplasmas may play an important regulatory role in HIV expression.

There is some preliminary evidence that mycoplasmal infections are associated with various autoimmune diseases. In some mycoplasma-positive GWI cases the signs and symptoms of Multiple Sclerosis (MS), Amyotrophic Lateral Sclerosis (ALS), Lupus, Graves' Disease and other complex autoimmune diseases have been seen. Such usually rare autoimmune responses are consistent with certain chronic infections, such as mycoplasmal infections, that penetrate into nerve cells, synovial cells and other cell types. The autoimmune signs and symptoms could be the result of intracellular pathogens, such as mycoplasmas, escaping from cellular compartments and incorporating into their own structures pieces of host cell membranes that contain important host antigens that can trigger autoimmune responses. Alternatively, mycoplasma surface components, sometimes called 'superantigens,' may directly stimulate autoimmune responses (43). Perhaps the most important event, the molecular mimicry of host antigens by mycoplasma surface components, may explain, in part, their ability to stimulate autoimmune responses (44).

Asthma, airway inflammation, chronic pneumonia and other respiratory diseases are known to be associated with mycoplasmal infections (45). For example, *M. pneumoniae* is a common cause of upper respiratory infections (46), and severe Asthma is frequently associated with mycoplasmal infections (47).

Cardiopathies can be caused by chronic infections, resulting in myocarditis, endocarditis, pericarditis and others. These are often due to chronic infections by *Mycoplasma* spp. (48), *Chlamydia* spp. (49) and possibly other infectious agents.

Mycoplasmal infections are also associated with a variety of illnesses, such as *M. hominis* infections in patients with hypogammaglobulinemia (29), and *M. genitalium* with nongonococcal urethritis (50). Mycoplasmas can exist in the oral cavity and gut as normal flora, but when they penetrate into the blood and tissues, they may be able to cause or promote a variety of acute or chronic illnesses. These cell-penetrating species, such as *M. penetrans, M. fermentans, M. hominis* and *M. pirum*, among others, can cause infections that result in complex systemic signs and symptoms. Mycoplasmal infections can also cause synergism with other infectious agents. Similar types of chronic infections caused by *Chlamydia, Brucella, Coxiella* or *Borriela* may also be present either as single agents or as complex, multiple infections in many chronic illnesses (9).

MYCOPLASMA TREATMENT

Although mycoplasmal infections are often misdiagnosed or inappropriately treated (45), they can be successfully treated using antibiotics and nutritional support (51,52). Appropriate treatment with antibiotics should result in patient improvement and even recovery, and this has been seen in GWI, CFS, FMS and RA patients (Table 2). The recommended treatments for mycoplasmal blood infections require long-term antibiotic therapy, usually 12 months or more or multiple 6-week cycles of doxycycline (200-300 mg/day), ciprofloxacin (1,500 mg/day), azithromycin (500 mg/day) or clarithromycin (750-1,000 mg/day). Multiple cycles are required, because only a few patients recovered after a few cycles, possibly because of the intracellular locations of pathogenic mycoplasmas, the slow-growing nature of

TABLE 2. Summary of chronic illness patients' antibiotic treatment results.

Percent Patients Mycoplasma-Positive or Responding to Therapy

Reference	(A)	(B)	(C)	(D)	(E)
Gulf War Illness (n)	(30)	(170)			
Blinded, controlled study (Y/N)	(No)	(No)			
Mycoplasma-positive pts	47	46			
Clinical Response*	ND	ND			
Clinical Recovery*	78	80			
CFS/FMS (n)			(30)		
Blinded, controlled study (Y/N)			(No)		
Mycoplasma-positive pts			66		
Clinical Response*			80		
Clinical Recovery*			50		
Rheumatoid Arthritis (n)				(219)	(46)
Blinded, controlled study (Y/N)				(Yes)	(Yes)
Mycoplasma-positive pts				ND	ND
Clinical Response				54	63
Clinical Recovery				ND	50

References: A, Nicolson and Nicolson, 1996 (15); B, Nicolson et al., 1998 (16); C, Nicolson, 1999 (53); D, Tilley et al., 1995 (34); (E), O'Dell et al., 1999 (55). *, Data only for mycoplasma-positive patients; ND, not determined.

these microorganisms and their relative drug sensitivities. For example, of 87 GWI patients that tested positive for mycoplasmal infections, all patients relapsed after the first 6-week cycle of antibiotic therapy, but after up to 6-7 cycles of therapy 69/87 patients responded and eventually recovered and returned to active duty (15,16) (Table 2). Similarly, the majority of CFS/FMS patients who tested positive for mycoplasmal infections also responded to the antibiotic therapy (53) (Table 2). Although these clinical studies were not placebo-controlled, blinded studies, double-blind, placebo-controlled antibiotic trials using minocycline versus placebo treatment of RA patients indicates that this antibiotic is clinically effective in RA (34,54) (Table 2).

The clinical responses that were seen in mycoplasma-positive chronic illness patients were not due to placebo effects, because administration of some antibiotics, such as penicillins, resulted in patients becoming more not less symptomatic, and they were not due to immunosuppressive effects that can occur with some of the recommended antibiotics (6,9,16). Interestingly, CFS, FMS and GWI patients that slowly recover after several cycles of antibiotics are generally less environmentally sensitive, suggesting that their immune systems may be returning to pre-illness states. If these illnesses were caused by psychological problems or solely by environmental exposures rather than infections, they should not respond to the recommended antibiotics and slowly recover. In addition, if such treatments were just reducing autoimmune responses, then patients should relapse after the treatments are discontinued, and this is not what has been found. CFS, FMS, RA or GWI patients also have nutritional and vitamin deficiencies that must be corrected (52,53). In addition, a fully functional immune system may be essential to overcoming these infections, and supplements and immune enhancers appear to be effective in helping patients recover (52,53).

Although we have proposed that chronic infections are an appropriate explanation for the morbidity seen in a rather large subset of CFS, FMS, GWI and RA patients, and in a variety of other chronic illnesses, not every patient will have this as a diagnostic explanation or have the same types of chronic infections. Additional research will be necessary to clarify the role of multiple infections in chronic diseases, but these patients could benefit from appropriate antibiotic and neutraceutical therapies that alleviate morbidity.

REFERENCES

1. Morrison, J.D. Fatigue as a presenting complaint in family practice. *Journal of Family Practice* 1980; 10: 795-801.

2. Kroenke, K., Wood, D.R., Mangelsdorff, A.D. et al. Chronic fatigue in primary care. Prevalence, patient characteristics and outcome. *JAMA* 1988; 260: 929-934.

3. Fukuda, K., Straus, S., Hickie, I., et al. The Chronic Fatigue Syndrome: a comprehensive approach to its definition and study. *Annuals of Internal Medicine* 1994; 121: 953-959.

4. Buchwald, D. and Garrity, D. Chronic fatigue, fibromyalgia and chemical sensitivity: overlapping disorders. *Archives of Internal Medicine* 1994; 154: 2049-2053.

5. Nicolson, G.L. and Nicolson, N.L. Chronic Fatigue illness and Operation Desert Storm. *Journal of Occupational and Environmental Medicine* 1995; 38: 14-17.

6. Nicolson, G.L., Nasralla, M., Haier, J. et al. Diagnosis and treatment of mycoplasmal infections in Fibromyalgia and Chronic Fatigue Syndromes: relationship to Gulf War Illness. *Biomedical Therapy* 1998; 16: 266-271.

7. Klimas, N. Salvato, F., Morgan, R. et al. Immunologic abnormalities in chronic fatigue syndrome. *Journal of Clinical Microbiology* 1990: 28: 1403-1410.

8. Dunn, A.J., Wang, J. and Ando, T. Effects of cytokines on cerebral neurotransmission. Comparison with the effects of stress. *Advances in Experimental Medicine and Biology* 1999; 461: 117-127.

9. Nicolson, G.L., Nasralla, M.Y., Haier, J. et al. Mycoplasmal infections in chronic illnesses: Fibromyalgia and Chronic Fatigue Syndromes, Gulf War Illness, HIV-AIDS and Rheumatoid Arthritis. *Medical Sentinel* 1999: 5: 172-176.

10. Nicolson, G.L. Chronic infections as a common etiology for many patients with Chronic Fatigue Syndrome, Fibromyalgia Syndrome and Gulf War Illnesses. *Intern. Journal of Medicine* 1998; 1: 42-46.

11. Hoffman, C., Rice, D. and Sung, H.-Y. Persons with chronic conditions. Their prevalence and costs. *JAMA* 1996; 276: 1473-1479.

12. Arnet, F.C., Edworthy S.M., Bloch, D.A., McShane, D.J., Fries, J.F., Cooper, N.S., et al. The American Rheumatism Association 1987 revised criteria for the classification of rheumatoid arthritis. *Arthritis Rheumatol* 1988; 31: 315-324.

13. Haier, J., Nasralla, M., Franco, A.R. and Nicolson, G.L. Detection of mycoplasmal infections in the blood of patients with Rheumatoid Arthritis. *Rheumatology* 1999; 38: 504-509.

14. Baseman, J.B. and Tully, J.G. Mycoplasmas: sophisticated, re-emerging and burdened by their notoriety. *Emerging Infectious Diseases* 1997; 3: 21-32.

15. Nicolson, G.L. and Nicolson, N.L. Diagnosis and treatment of mycoplasmal infections in Persian Gulf War Illness-CFIDS patients. *Intern. Journal of Occupational Medicine, Immunology and Toxicology* 1996; 5: 69-78.

16. Nicolson, G.L., Nicolson, N.L. and Nasralla, M. Mycoplasmal infections and Chronic Fatigue Illness (Gulf War Illness) associated with deployment to Operation Desert Storm. *International Journal of Medicine* 1998; 1: 80-92.

17. Nasralla, M., Haier, J. and Nicolson, G.L. Multiple mycoplasmal infections detected in blood of Chronic Fatigue and Fibromyalgia Syndrome patients. *European Journal of Clinical Microbiology and Infectious Diseases* 1999; 18:859-865.

18. Erlich, H. A., Gelfand, D. and Sninsky, J. J. Recent advances in the polymerase chain reaction. *Science* 1991; 252: 1643-1651.

19. Vojdani, A., Choppa, P.C., Tagle, C., Andrin, R., Samimi, B. and Lapp, C.W. Detection of *Mycoplasma* genus and *Mycoplasma fermentans* by PCR in patients with Chronic Fatigue Syndrome. *FEMS Immunology and Medical Microbiology* 1998; 22: 355-365.

20. Huang, W., See, D. and Tiles, J. The prevalence of *Mycoplasma incognitus* in the peripheral blood mononuclear cells of normal controls or patients with AIDS or Chronic Fatigue Syndrome. *Journal of Chronic Fatigue Syndrome* 1999; in press.

21. Choppa, Vojdani, A., Tagle, C., Andrin, R. and Magtoto, L. Multiplex PCR for the detection of *Mycoplasma fermentans*, *M. hominis* and *M. penetrans* in cell cultures and blood samples of patients with Chronic Fatigue Syndrome. *Molecular and Cellular Probes* 1998; 12: 301-308.

22. Vojdani, A. and Franco, A.R. Multiplex PCR for the detection of *Mycoplasma fermentans*, *M. hominis* and *M. penetrans* in patients with Chronic Fatigue Syndrome, Fibromyalgia, Rheumatoid Arthritis and Gulf War Illness. *Journal of Chronic Fatigue Syndrome* 1999; 5: 187-197.

23. Nasralla, M.Y., Haier, J. and Nicolson, G.L. Determination of mycoplasmal infections in blood of 565 Chronic Fatigue Syndrome and Fibromyalgia Syndrome patients detected by polymerase chain reaction (submitted).

24. Krause, A., Samradt, T. and Burnmester, G.R. Potential infectious agents in the induction of arthritides. *Current Opinion of Rheumatology* 1996; 8: 203-209.

25. Midvedt, T. Intestinal bacteria and rheumatic disease. *Scandinavian Journal of Rheumatology Suppl.* 1987; 64: 49-54.

26. Fox, R.I., Luppi, M., Pisa, P. et al. Potential role of Epstein-Bar virus in Sjögren's syndrome and rheumatoid arthritis. *Journal of Rheumatology* 1992; 32(Suppl): 18-24.

27. Tsai, Y.T., Chiang, B.L., Kao, Y.F. et al. Detection of Epstein-Bar virus and cytomegalovirus genome in white blood cells from patients with juvenile rheumatoid arthritis and childhood systemic lupus erythematosus. *Intern. Archives of Allergy and Immunology* 1995; 106: 235-240.

28. Schaeverbeke, T., Renaudin, H. Clerc, M. et al. Systematic detection of myco-plasmas by culture and polymerase chain reaction (PCR) procedures in 209 synovial fluid samples. *Reviews Rheumatology* 1997; 64: 120-128.

29. Furr, P.M., Taylor-Robinson, D. and Webster, A.D.B. Mycoplasmas and urea-plasmas in patients with hypogammaglobulinemia and their roll in arthritis: microbi-ological observation over twenty years. *Annuals of Rheumatological Diseases* 1994; 53: 183-187.

30. Simecka, J.W., Ross, S.E., Cassell, G.H. and Davis, J.K. Interactions of myco-plasmas with B cells: production of antibodies and nonspecific effects. *Clinical Infectious Diseases* 1993; 17 (Supp. 1): S176-S182.

31. Cole, B.C. and Griffith, M.M. Triggering and exacerbation of auroimmune ar-thritis by the *Mycoplasma arthritidis* superantigen MAM. *Arthritis and Rheumatolo-gy* 1993; 36: 994-1002.

32. Kirchhoff, H., Binder, A., Runge, M. et al. Pathogenic mechanisms in the *My-coplasma arthritidis* polyarthritis of rats. *Rheumatology Int.* 1989; 9: 193-196.

33. Mühlradt, P.F., Quentmeier, H. and Schmitt, E. Involvement of interleukin-1 (IL-1), IL-6, IL-2 and IL-4 in generation of cytolytic T cells from thymocytes stimu-lated by a *Mycoplasma fermentans*-derived product. *Infection and Immunology* 1991; 58: 1273-1280.

34. Tilley, B.C., Alarcon, G.S., Heyse, S.P. et al. Minocycline in rheumatoid ar-thritis. A 48-week, double-blind, placebo-controlled trial. *Annuals of Internal Medi-cine* 1995: 122: 81-89.

35. Hawkins, R.E., Rickman, L.S., Vermund, S.H. et al. Association of *Mycoplas-ma* and human immunodeficiency virus infection: detection of amplified *Mycoplas-ma fermentans* DNA in blood. *Journal of Infectious Diseases* 1992; 165: 581-585.

36. Lo, S.-C., Dawson, M.S., Newton, P.B. et al. Association of the virus-like in-fectious agent originally reported in patients with AIDS with acute fatal disease in previously healthy non-AIDS patients. *American Journal of Tropical Medicine and Hygiene* 1989; 41: 364-376.

37. Blanchard, A. and Montagnier, L. AIDS associated mycoplasmas. *Annual Re-view of Microbiology* 1994; 48: 687-712.

38. Bauer, F.A., Wear, D.J., Angritt, P. and Lo, S.-C. *Mycoplasma fermentans* (incognitus strain) infection in the kidneys of patients with acquired immunodefi-ciency syndrome and associated nephropathy: a light microscopic, immunohis-tochemical and ultrastructural study. *Human Pathology* 1991; 22, 63-69.

39. Sloot, N., Hollandt, H. Gatermann, S. and Dalhoff, K. Detection of *Mycoplasma* spp. in bronchoalveolar lavage of AIDS patients with pulmonary infiltrates. *Zentralbl Bacteriology* 1996; 284: 75-79.

40. Grau, O., Slizewicz, B. Tuppin, P. et al. Association of *Mycoplasma penetrans* with human immunodeficiency virus infection. *Journal of Infectious Disease* 1995; 172: 672-681.

41. Pollack, J.D., Jones, M.A. and Williams, M.V. The metabolism of ADIS-associated mycoplasmas. *Clinical Infectious Diseases* 1993; 17: S267-S271.

42. Nir-Paz, R., Israel, S., Honigman, A. and Kahane, I. Mycoplasmas regulate HIV-LTR-dependent gene expression. *FEMS Microbiology Letters* 1995; 128: 63-68.

43. Kaneoka, H. and Naito, S. Superantigens and autoimmune diseases. *Japanese Journal of Clinical Medicine* 1997; 6: 1363-1369.

44. Dallo, S.F., Lazzell, A.L., Charoya, A., Reddy, S.P., and Baseman, J.B. Biofunctional domains of the *Mycoplasma pneumoniae* P30 adhesion. *Infect Immun* 1996; 64(7): 2595-2601.

45. Cassell, G.H. Infectious causes of chronic inflammatory diseases and cancer. *Emerging Infectious Diseases* 1998; 4: 475-487.

46. Kraft, M., Cassell, G.H., Henson, J.E. et al. Detection of *Mycoplasma pneumoniae* in the airways of adults with chronic asthma. *American Journal of Respiratory Critical Care Medicine* 1998; 158: 998-1001.

47. Gil, J.C., Cedillo, R.L., Mayagoitia, B.G. and Paz, M.D. Isolation of *Mycoplasma pneumoniae* from asthmatic patients. *Annuals of Allergy* 1993; 70: 23-25.

48. Prattichizzo, F.A., Simonetti, I. and Galetta, F. Carditis associated with *Mycoplasma pneumoniae* infections. Clinical aspects and therapeutic problems. *Minerva Cardioangiology* 1997; 45: 447-450.

49. Fairley, C.K.l, Ryan, M., Wall, P.G. and Weinberg, J. The organisms reported to cause infective myocarditis and pericarditis in England and Wales. *Journal of Infection* 1996; 32: 223-225.

50. Busolo, F., Camposampiero, D., Bordignon, G. and Bertollo, G. Detection of *Mycoplasma genitalium* and *Chlamydia trachomatis* DNAs in male patients with urethritis using the polymerase chain reaction. *New Microbiologia* 1997; 20: 325-332.

51. Nicolson, G.L. and Nicolson, N.L. Doxycycline treatment and Desert Storm. *JAMA* 1996; 273: 618-619.

52. Nicolson, G.L. Considerations when undergoing treatment for chronic infections found in Chronic Fatigue Syndrome, Fibromyalgia Syndrome and Gulf War Illnesses. (Part 1). Antibiotics Recommended when indicated for treatment of Gulf War Illness/CFIDS/FMS (Part 2). *Intern. Journal of Medicine* 1998; 1: 115-117, 123-128.

53. Nicolson, G.L. The role of microorganism infections in chronic illnesses: support for antibiotic regimens. *CFIDS Chronicle* 1999; 12(3): 19-21.

54. O'Dell, J.R., Paulsen, G. Haire, C.E. et al. Treatment of early seropositive rheumatoid arthritis with minocycline: four-year follow-up of a double-blind, placebo-controlled trial. *Arthritis and Rheumatology* 1999; 42: 1691-1695.

Human Herpes Virus 6 (HHV-6) Infection in Patients with Chronic Fatigue Syndrome and Its Relationship to Activation-Induced Cell Death

Alan M. Cocchetto, MS
Mary E. McNamara, MBA
Edward F. Jordan, MD

SUMMARY. Using evidence-based medical research techniques, current knowledge about the presence of active HHV-6 infections, in a sub-population of patients with chronic fatigue syndrome (CFS), has been reviewed and implications to activation-induced cell death are presented. Therapeutic intervention methods are also disclosed with a call for clinical studies to test the hypothesis presented. *[Article copies available for a fee from The Haworth Document Delivery Service: 1-800-342-9678. E-mail address: <getinfo@haworthpressinc.com> Website: <http://www.haworthpressinc. com>]*

KEYWORDS. Human herpes virus 6 (HHV-6), activation-induced cell death, chronic fatigue syndrome

---

Alan M. Cocchetto is Associate Professor of Electrical Engineering Technology, Alfred State College, SUNY at Alfred, Alfred, NY 14802 and is Medical Advisor for the National CFIDS Foundation, Inc., Needham, MA 02492.

Mary E. McNamara is Vice President and Director of Research of the New Jersey Chronic Fatigue Syndrome Association, Inc., Chatham, NJ 07928.

Edward F. Jordan is Internist and Oncologist who maintains a private practice in Olean, NY 14760.

Address correspondence to: Profesor Alan M. Cocchetto, 1113 Sharps Hill Road, Arkport, NY 14807 (E-mail: cocc1113@linkny.com).

[Haworth co-indexing entry note]: "Human Herpes Virus 6 (HHV-6) Infection in Patients with Chronic Fatigue Syndrome and Its Relationship to Activation-Induced Cell Death." Cocchetto, Alan M., Mary E. McNamara, and Edward F. Jordan. Co-published simultaneously in *Journal of Chronic Fatigue Syndrome* (The Haworth Medical Press, an imprint of The Haworth Press, Inc.) Vol. 6, No. 3/4, 2000, pp. 41-50; and: *Chronic Fatigue Syndrome: Critical Reviews and Clinical Advances* (ed: Kenny De Meirleir, and Roberto Patarca-Montero) The Haworth Medical Press, an imprint of The Haworth Press, Inc., 2000, pp. 41-50. Single or multiple copies of this article are available for a fee from The Haworth Document Delivery Service [1-800-342-9678, 9:00 a.m. - 5:00 p.m. (EST). E-mail address: getinfo@haworthpressinc.com].

Since the Lake Tahoe outbreak, human herpesvirus-6 (HHV-6) infection has been reported to be associated with chronic fatigue syndrome (CFS) (1). Numerous publications have suggested that more than a casual relationship exists between HHV-6 infection and the development of CFS (2-18).

Human herpesvirus-6, previously known as HBLV, is a T-lymphotropic beta-herpesvirus which has two variants, A and B (19,20). Known to be a very destructive virus (21), HHV-6 can cause severe immunosuppression by killing CD4+ as well as CD8+ T-lymphocytes (22,23) and natural killer NK cells (24), and it can induce high levels of pro-inflammatory cytokines (25,26). The direct immunosuppressive effects of HHV-6 have been shown to directly alter these critical T-cell components in a patient with chronic fatigue syndrome using serial lymphocyte subtype monitoring (27). Cellular proliferation is adversely affected by the alteration of growth factors by HHV-6 as well (28). One unusual but intriguing characteristic of HHV-6 variant A infected cells is the virtual absence of viral glycoproteins on their plasma membrane (29). Also, it is important to note the clinical comparisons, regarding T-cell immune activation profiles of CD8+ cells showing HLA-DR and CD38 markers, between HIV and chronic fatigue syndrome patients (30-33).

Numerous diseases have been associated with HHV-6 in both immunosuppressed and immunocompetent hosts (34). HHV-6 has been associated with multiple sclerosis (35-37). Due to its destructive nature, HHV-6 has also been suggested as a cofactor in AIDS (13,38-43). HHV-6 infection may predispose cells to superinfection by other viruses (44). HHV-6 has been shown to be synergistic with Epstein-Barr virus (EBV) (45,46). Ironically, a similar association exists between EBV and HIV (47). Likewise, associations between chronic fatigue syndrome and cancer have also raised suspicions in the medical community (48,49). HHV-6 has associations with cancer as well (50-52).

HHV-6 appears to have a dual personality based on the variant involved and results so far available support the hypothesis that HHV-6 variants may have different epidemiologies (53). It has been suspected that HHV-6A is more immunotropic while HHV-6B is more neurotropic because variant A is seen in immmunocompromised patients while variant B is associated with exanthema subitum (roseola infantum), a febrile disorder (13).

It has been shown that HHV-6 transcriptionally downregulates the expression of CD3 (22). Because activated T-cells are involved in this downregulation, there is an alteration of the T-cell receptor TCR/CD3 complex. The resulting immunosuppression, due to this down-regulation, has been studied by various scientists (54,55) and it has been determined that mature T-cells are the key target for destruction.

Because persistent infection with HHV-6 could provide prolonged stimulation to T-cells, this would render them susceptible to activation-induced cell death (AICD) which would greatly accelerate the apoptotic or cell death mechanism directly in these cells. This is an intriguing concept since CFS patients are known to have accentuated apoptosis levels (56,57) as well as altered levels of B-cell lymphoma/leukemia-2 (bcl-2) expression (58).

CD95, also referred to as Fas or APO-1, is an important receptor in apoptosis. Apoptotic cell death is triggered by an interaction of the CD95 receptor with its ligand CD95L (59). The CD95 ligand is a transmembrane molecule of the tumor necrosis factor (TNF) family that is produced by activated T-cells and is constitutively expressed in a variety of tissues. It has been reported that CD95L expression may provide a mechanism of immune privilege in several anatomical sites and tumors (60-63). Thus, T-cells may become blindfolded to attack the respective tissues (64). TCR triggering in activated T-cells may induce apoptosis involving autocrine suicide or paracrine death mediated via CD95 receptor/ligand interaction (65,66). Expression of CD95 contributes to the physiological growth control as well as to the pathology of increased cell death that is seen in AIDS (67,68), EBV infections (69), cytomegalovirus (CMV) infections (70), HTLV-1 infections (71), and perhaps in CFS patients with HHV-6 infections as well. Likewise, induction of this ligand could cause accelerated apoptosis in T-cells thereby diminishing their numbers and producing subsequent immunosuppression in the host leaving it susceptible to opportunistic infections.

Recent evidence suggests that bcl-2 proteins modify the cell death program (72) via their influence on mitochondrial function as well as their control over activation of cysteine proteases of the caspase family (73,74). The caspases are considered to be the cell death executioners due to the absolute requirements for their presence in cell death (64). Likewise, inhibition of the function of caspases is generally associated with the inhibition of cell death. Perhaps the increased levels of bcl-2, found in CFS patients (58), is a means for the body to adjust for increasing apoptosis levels. However, this could prove to be potentially dangerous in patients who have HHV-6 as well as EBV infections, since the overexpression of bcl-2 may provide a step towards B-cell immortalization and transformation through an inappropriate prolongation of infected cell survival (75).

It has been shown that dendritic cells (DC), which are highly effective antigen-presenting cells (APC), prevent T-cell apoptosis (76). Dendritic cells prevent CD95/Fas-triggered apoptosis by inhibiting the activation of caspase 8 and caspase 3 (77). It has also been shown that since this protective effect of the dendritic cells on T-cell death could be blocked by anti-CD58 antibodies, CD58 ligation plays a key role in this process (76). Fortunately, scientists have shown that the lipoxygenase inhibitor, nordihydroguaiaretic acid (NDGA), inhibits caspase 8 and caspase 3 activation and acts to reduce apoptosis (78). Furthermore, bcl-2, crm-A, and NDGA have been shown to act upstream of the caspases to inhibit apoptosis.

Tied also to the CD95/Fas/APO-1 pathway are glutathione levels. Glutathione levels are important in antigen-presenting cells because they act as a key regulatory element in the process of modulating T helper 1 (Th1) and T helper 2 (Th2) cytokine response patterns that are fundamental to the immune response (79). Th1 and Th2 responses are involved in the cell mediated and humoral mediated immune responses respectively. In AIDS, glutathione deficiency is associated with impaired survival in HIV disease (80) and the use of N-acetyl cysteine (NAC), orally administered, improved patient survival (81,82). Likewise, the overexpression of bcl-2, crm-A, or the use of N-acetyl cysteine confers resistance to apoptosis mediated by TNF-alpha in HIV (83).

The significance of these pathways, molecular expressions, and corresponding drug modulators should prove to be vitally important to the patient's health. Therefore, the use of these types of agents should prove to be restorative to T cells due to the near normalization of apoptotic levels and thus serve to ameliorate inappropriate cellular activation thereby assisting the host in fighting HHV-6 infection. As a result, NDGA, N-acetyl cysteine and other similar inhibitors should prove to be critically useful in reducing activation induced cell death in T cells. Specific studies with CFS patients having active HHV-6 Variant A infections should serve as a starting point for investigational work to solidify this hypothesis especially given the availability of the modifying agents.

REFERENCES

1. Barnes DM. Mystery disease at Lake Tahoe challenges virologists and clinicians. *Science.* 1986;234:541-542.

2. Ablashi DV, Zompetta C, Lease C, Josephs SF, Balachandran N, Komaroff AL, Krueger GR, Henry B, Lukau J, Salahuddin SZ. Human herpesvirus 6 (HHV-6) and chronic fatigue syndrome. *Canad Dis Weekly Rep.* 1991;17S1E;33-41.

3. Komaroff AL. Human herpesvirus-6 and human disease. *Am J Clin Pathol.* 1990;93(6):836-837.

4. Josephs SF, Henry B, Balachandran N, Strayer D, Peterson D, Komaroff AL, Ablashi DV. HHV-6 reactivation in chronic fatigue syndrome [letter]. *Lancet.* 1991; 337:1346-1347.

5. Buchwald D, Cheney PR, Peterson DL, Henry B, Wormsley SB, Geiger A, Ablashi DV, Salahuddin SZ, Saxinger C, Biddle R, Kikinis R, Jolesz FA, Folks T, Balachandran N, Peter JB, Gallo RC, Komaroff AL. A chronic illness characterized by fatigue, neurologic and immunologic disorders, and active human herpesvirus type 6 infection. *Ann Intern Med.* 1992;116:103-113.

6. Krueger GR, Klueppelberg U, Hoffman A, Ablashi DV. Clinical correlates of infection with human herpesvirus-6. *InVivo.* 1994;8:457-486.

7. Yalcin S, Kuratsune H, Yamaguchi K, Kitani T, Yamanishi K. Prevalence of human herpesvirus 6 variants A and B in patients with chronic fatigue syndrome. *Microbiol Immunol.* 1994;38:587-590.

8. DiLuca D, Zorzenon M, Mirandola P, Colle R, Botta GA, Cassai E. Human herpesvirus 6 and human herpesvirus 7 in chronic fatigue syndrome. *J Clin Microbiol.* 1995;33:1660-1661.

9. Patnaik M, Komaroff AL, Conley E, Ojo-Amaize E, Peter JB. Prevalence of IgM antibodies to human herpesvirus 6 early antigen (p41/38) in patients with chronic fatigue syndrome. *J Infect Dis.* 1995;172:1364-1367.

10. Strayer DR, Carter W, Strauss K, Brodsky I, Suhadolnik R, Ablashi DV, Henry B, Mitchell WM, Bastien S, Peterson D. Long term improvements in patients with chronic fatigue syndrome treated with ampligen. *Journal of Chronic Fatigue Syndrome.* 1995;1(1):35-53.

11. Ablashi DV, Ablashi K, Kramarsky B, Bernbaum J, Whitman JE, Pearson GR. Viruses and chronic fatigue syndrome: current status. *Journal of Chronic Fatigue Syndrome.* 1995;1(1):3-22.

12. Levine PH. A review of human herpesvirus 6 infections. *Infections in Medicine.* 1995;395-402.

13. Lusso P. Human herpesvirus 6 (HHV-6) [Mini-review]. *Antiviral Research.* 1996;31:1-21.

14. Zorzenon M, Rukh G, Botta G, Colle R, Barrsanti L, Ceccherini-Nelli L. Active HHV-6 infection in chronic fatigue syndrome patients from Italy: new data. *Journal of Chronic Fatigue Syndrome.* 1996;2(1):3-12.

15. Wagner M, Krueger GRF, Ablashi DV, Whitman JE. Chronic fatigue syndrome (CFS): a critical evaluation of testing for active human herpesvirus-6 (HHV-6) infection: review of data of 107 cases. *Journal of Chronic Fatigue Syndrome.* 1996; 2(4):3-16.

16. Salahuddin SZ, Ablashi DV, Josephs SF, Saxinger CW, Wong-Staal F, Gallo RC, inventors; The Government of the United States of America, assignee. Human herpesvirus-6 (HHV-6) isolution and products. US patent 5 604 093. February 18, 1997.

17. Knox KK, Brewer JH, Carrigan DR. Persistent Active human herpesvirus six (HHV-6) infections in patients with chronic fatigue syndrome. In: Proceedings of the AACFS Fourth International Research, Clinical and Patient Conference on Chronic Fatigue Syndrome; October 10-12, 1998; Cambridge, MA.

18. Ablashi DV, Marsh S, Handy M, Whitman J, Viza D, Krueger GR, Levine PH. Increased activation of human herpesvirus-6 (HHV-6), but not human herpesvirus-7 (HHV-7) or human herpesvirus-8 (HHV-8), in chronic fatigue syndrome (CFS) patients. In: Proceedings of the AACFS Fourth International Research, Clinical and Patient Conference on Chronic Fatigue Syndrome; October 10-12, 1998; Cambridge, MA.

19. Salahuddin SZ, Ablashi DV, Markham PD, Josephs SF, Sturzenegger S, Kaplan M, Halligan G, Bibberfeld P, Wong-Staal F, Kramarsky B, Gallo RC. Isolation of a new virus, HBLV, in patients with lymphoproliferative disorders. *Science.* 1986;234:596-601.

20. Dockrell DH, Smith TF, Paya CV. Human herpesvirus 6. *Mayo Clin Proc.* 1999;74:163-170.

21. Ablashi DV, Balachandran N, Josephs SF, Hung CL, Krueger GR, Kramarsky B, Salahuddin SZ, Gallo RC. Genomic polymorphism, growth properties, and immunologic variations in human herpesvirus 6 isolates. *Virology.* 1991;184(2):545-552.

22. Lusso P, Malnati M, DeMaria A, Balotta C, DeRocco SE, Markham PD, Gallo RC. Productive infection of CD4+ and CD8+ mature T-cell populations and clones by HHV-6: transcriptional down-regulation of CD3. *J Immunol.* 1991;147(2):685-691.

23. Knox KK, Pietryga D, Harrington DJ, Franciosi R, Carrigan DR. Progressive immunodeficiency and fatal pneumonitis associated with HHV-6 infection in an infant. *Clin Infect Dis.*1995;20:406-413.

24. Lusso P, Malnati MS, Garzino-Demo A, Crowley RW, Long EO, Gallo RC. Infection of natural killer cells by human herpesvirus 6. *Nature.* 1993;362:458-462.

25. Flamand L, Gosselin J, D'Addario M, Hiscott J, Ablashi DV, Gallo RC, Menezes J. Human herpesvirus 6 induces interleukin-1B and tumor necrosis factor alpha, but not interleukin-6 in peripheral blood mononuclear cell cultures. *J Virol.* 1991;65:5105-5110.

26. Gosselin J, Flamand L, D'Addario M, Hiscott J, Stefanescu I, Ablashi DV, Gallo RC, Menezes J. Modulatory effects of Epstein-Barr, herpes simplex and human herpesvirus 6 viral infections and coinfections on cytokine synthesis: a comparative study. *J Immunol.* 1992;149:181-187.

27. Krueger G, Koch B, Ablashi DV. Persistent fatigue and depression in patient with antibody to human B-lymphotropic virus. *Lancet.* 1987;2(8549):36.

28. Flamand L, Gosselin J, Stefanescu I, Ablashi DV, Menezes J. Immunosuppressive effect of human herpesvirus 6 on T-cell functions: suppression of interleukin-2 synthesis and cell proliferation. *Blood.* 1995;85(5):1263-1271.

29. Torrisi MR, Gentile M, Cardinali G, Cirone M, Zompetta C, Lotti LV, Frati L, Faggioni A. Intracellular transport and maturation pathway of human herpesvirus 6. *Virology.* 1999;257:460-471.

30. Landay AL, Jessop C, Lennette ET, Levy JA. Chronic fatigue syndrome: clinical condition associated with immune activation. *Lancet.* 1991;338(8769):707-712.

31. Giorgi JV, Hultin L, inventors; The Regents of the University of California, assignee. Method for determining favorable prognosis in an HIV positive subject using HLA-DR+ CD38-bright cells. US patent 5 470 701. November 28, 1995.

32. Levy JA, Landay AL, inventors; The Regents of the University of California, assignee. Screening kit and method for diagnosing chronic immune dysfunction syndrome. US patent 5 538 856. July 23, 1996.

33. Giorgi JV, Hultin LE, McKeating JA, Johnson TD, Owens B, Jacobson LP, Shih R, Lewis J, Wiley DC, Phair JP, Wolinsky SM, Detels R. Shorter survival in advanced human immunodeficiency virus type 1 infection is more closely associated with T lymphocyte activation than with plasma virus burden or virus chemokine coreceptor usage. *J Infect Dis.* 1999;179:859-870.

34. Caserta MT, Hall CB. Human herpesvirus-6. In: Scheld WM, Whiteley RJ, Durack DT, eds. *Infections of the Central Nervous Sytem.* 2nd ed. Philadelphia, PA: Lippincott-Raven Publishers;1997:129-138.

35. Challoner PB, Smith KT, Parker JD, MacLeod DL, Coulter SN, Rose TM, Schultz ER, Bennett JL, Garber RL, Chang M, Schad PA, Stewart PM, Nowinski RC, Brown JP, Burmer GC. Plaque associated expression of human herpesvirus 6 in multiple sclerosis. *Proc Natl Acad Sci.* 1995;2:7440-7444.

36. Carrigan DR, Knox KK. Human herpesvirus six and multiple sclerosis. *Multiple Sclerosis.* 1997;3(6):390-394.

37. Ablashi DV, Lapps W, Kaplan M, Whitman JE, Richert JR, Pearson GR. Human herpesvirus (HHV-6) infection in multiple sclerosis: a preliminary report. *Multiple Sclerosis.* 1998;4:490-496.

38. Lusso P, Markham PD, Ranki A, Earl P, Moss B, Donner F, Gallo RC, Krohn KJ. Cell-mediated immune response toward viral envelope and core antigens in gibbon apes (Hylobates lar) chronically infected with human immunodeficiency virus-1. *J Immunol.* 1988;141(7):2467-73.

39. Lusso P, Gallo RC. Human herpesvirus 6 in AIDS. *Immun Today.* 1995;16(2): 67-71.

40. Knox KK. *Human Herpesvirus Six (HHV-6): Evidence for Its Role as a Cofactor in the Pathogenesis of AIDS* [dissertation]. Milwaukee, WI: Medical College of Wisconsin; 1994.

41. Knox KK, Carrigan DR. Active HHV-6 infection in the lymph nodes of HIV-infected patients: *in vitro* evidence that HHV-6 can break HIV latency. *J Acquir Immune Defic Syndr Hum Retrovirol.* 1996;11(4):370-378.

42. Lusso P, Gallo RC. Human herpesvirus-6 in AIDS. *Lancet.* 1994;343:555-556.

43. Knox KK, Carrigan DR. Active human herpesvirus-6 (HHV-6) infection of the central nervous system in patients with AIDS. *J Acquir Immune Defic Syndr Hum Retrovirol.* 1995;9:69-73.

44. Schonnebeck M, Krueger GR, Braun M, Fischer M, Koch B, Ablashi DV, Balachandran N. Human herpesvirus-6 infection may predispose cells to superinfection by other viruses. *In Vivo.* 1991;5(3):255-263.

45. Flamand L, Stefanescu I, Ablashi DV, Menezes J. Activation of the Epstein-Barr virus replicative cycle by human herpesvirus 6. *J Virol.* 1993;67(11):6768-6777.

46. Cuomo L, Angeloni A, Zompetta C, Cirone M, Calogers A, Frati L, Ragona G, Faggioni A. Human herpesvirus 6 variant A, but not variant B, infects EBV-positive B lymphoid cells, activating the latent EBV genome through a BZLF-1-dependent mechanism. *AIDS Res Hum Retroviruses.* 1995;11:1241-1245.

47. Lynne J, Schmid I, Matud JL, Hirji K, Buessow S, Shlian DM, Giorgi JV. Major expansions of select CD8+ subsets in acute Epstein-Barr virus infection: comparison with chronic human immunodeficiency virus disease. *J Infect Dis.* 1998;177: 1083-1087

48. Levine PH, Fears TR, Cummings P, Hoover RN. Cancer and a fatiguing illness in Northern Nevada–a causal hypothesis. *Ann. Epidemiol.* 1998;8(4):245-249.

49. Levine PH, Whiteside TL, Friberg D, Bryant J, Colclough G, Herberman RB. Dysfunction of natural killer activity in a family with chronic fatigue syndrome. *Clin Immunol Immunopathol.* 1998;88(1):96-104.

50. Josephs SF, Buchbinder A, Streicher HZ, Ablashi DV, Salahuddin SZ, Guo HG, Wong-Staal F, Cossman J, Raffeld M, Sundeen J et al. Detection of human B-lymphotropic virus (human herpesvirus 6) sequences in B cell lymphoma tissues of three patients. *Leukemia* 1988;2(3):132-135.

51. Jarrett RF, Gledhill S, Qureshi F, Crae SH, Madhok R, Brown I, Evans I, Krajewski A, O'Brien CJ, Cartwright RA et al. Identification of human herpesvirus 6-specific DNA sequences in two patients with non-Hodgkin's lymphoma. *Leukemia.* 1988;2(8):496-502.

52. Yaddav M, Chandrashekran A, Vasudevan DM, Ablashi DV. Frequent detection of human herpesvirus-6 in oral carcinoma. *J Nat'l Cancer Institute.* 1994; 86(23):1792-1794.

53. DiLuca D, Mirandola P, Ravaioli T, Bigoni B, Cassai E. Distribution of HHV-6 variants in human tissues. *Infect Agents Dis.* 1996;5(4):203-214.

54. Kikuta H, Lu H, Tomizawa K, Matsumoto S. Enhancement of human herpesvirus 6 replication in adult human lymphocytes by monoclonal antibody to CD3. *J Infect Dis.* 1990;161:1085-1087.

55. Takahashi K, Sonoda S, Higashi K, Kondo T, Takahashi H, Takahashi M, Yamanishi K. Predominant CD4 T-lymphocyte tropism of human herpesvirus 6 related virus. *J Virol.* 1989;63:3161-3163.

56. Vojdani A, Ghoneum M, Choppa PC, Magtoto L, Lapp CW. Elevated apoptotic cell population in patients with chronic fatigue syndrome: the pivotal role of protein kinase RNA. *J Intern Med.* 1997;242(6):465-478.

57. See DM, Cimoch P, Chou S, Chang J, Tilles J. The *in vitro* immunomodulatory effects of glyconutrients on peripheral blood mononuclear cells of patients with chronic fatigue syndrome. *Integr Physiol Behav Sci.* 1998;33(3):280-287.

58. Hassan IS, Bannister BA, Akbar A, Weir W, Bofill M. A study of the immunology of the chronic fatigue syndrome: correlation of immunologic parameters to health dysfunction. *Clin Immunol Immunopathol.* 1998;87(1):60-67.

59. Watson JD, Rudert F, inventors; Genesis Research and Development Corporation Limited, assignee. CD95 regulatory gene sequences. US patent 5 912 168. June 15, 1999.

60. Nagata S, Golstein P. The Fas death factor. *Science.* 1995;267:1449-1456.

61. Krammer PH, Dhein J, Walczak H, Behrmann I, Mariani S, Matiba B, Fath M, Daniel PT, Knipping E, Westendorp MO et al. The role of APO-1 mediated apoptosis in the immune system. *Immunol Rev.* 1994;142:175-191.

62. Suda T, Takahashi T, Golstein P, Nagata S. Molecular cloning and expression of the Fas ligand, a novel member of the tumor necrosis factor family. *Cell.* 1993;75:1169-1178.

63. Bellgrau D, Gold D, Selawry H, Moore J, Franzusoff A, Duke RC. A role for CD95 ligand in preventing graft rejection. *Nature.* 1995;377:630-632.

64. Debatin K. Cell death program. In: Degos L, Linch DC, Lowenberg B, eds. *Textbook of Malignant Haematology.* London UK: Martin Dunitz Ltd; 1999:153-164.

65. Dhein J, Walczak H, Baumler C, Debatin KM, Krammer PH. Autocrine T-cell suicide mediated by APO-1/Fas/CD95. *Nature.* 1995;373:438-441.

66. Strasser A. Death of a T cell. *Nature.* 1995;373:385-386.

67. Katsikis PD, Wunderlich ES, Smith CA, Herzenberg LA, Herzenberg LA. Fas antigen stimulation induces marked apoptosis of T lymphocytes in human immunodeficiency virus-infected individuals. *J Exp Med.* 1995;181(6):2029-2036.

68. Katsikis PD, Garcia-Ojeda ME, Torres-Roca JF, Tijoe IM, Smith CA, Herzenberg LA, Herzenberg LA. Interleukin-1 beta converting enzyme-like protease involvement in Fas-induced and activation-induced peripheral blood T cell apoptosis in HIV infection. TNF-related apoptosis-inducing ligand can mediate activation-induced T cell death in HIV infection. *J Exp Med.* 1997;186(8):1365-1372.

69. Larochelle B, Flamand L, Gourde P, Beauchamp D, Gosselin J. Epstein-Barr virus infects and induces apoptosis in human neutrophils. *Blood.* 1998;92(1):291-299.

70. Craigen JL, Grundy JE. Cytomegalovirus induced up-regulation of LFA-3 (CD58) and ICAM-1 (CD54) is a direct viral effect that is not prevented by ganciclovir or foscarnet treatment. *Transplantation.* 1996;62(8):1102-1108.

71. de Waal Malefyt R, Yssel H, Spits H, de Vries JE, Sancho J, Terhorst C, Alarcon B. Human T cell leukemia virus type 1 prevents cell surface expression of the T cell receptor through down-regulation of the CD3-gamma, -delta, -epsilon, and -zeta genes. *J Immunol.* 1990;145(7):2297-2303.

72. Strasser A, Harris AW, Huang DC, Krammer PH, Cory S. Bcl-2 and Fas/APO-1 regulate distinct pathways to lymphocyte apoptosis. *EMBO J.* 1995;14(24):6136-6147.

73. Kroemer G. The proto-oncogene bcl-2 and its role in regulating apoptosis. *Nature Med.* 1997;3:614-620.

74. Reed JC. Double identity for proteins of the Bcl-2 family. *Nature.* 1997;387:773-776.

75. Lyons SF, Liebowitz DN. The roles of human viruses in the pathogenesis of lymphoma. *Sem in Oncology* 1998;25(4):461-475.

76. Daniel PT, Scholz C, Essmann F, Westermann J, Dorken B, Pezzutto A. Dendritic cells prevent CD95 mediated T lymphocyte death through costimulatory signals. *Adv Exp Med Biol.* 1998;451:173-177.

77. Daniel PT, Scholz C, Essmann F, Westermann J, Pezzutto A, Dorken B. CD95/Fas-triggered apoptosis of activated T lymphocytes is prevented by dendritic cells through a CD58-dependent mechanism. *Exp Hematol.* 1999;27(9):1402-1408.

78. Wagenknecht B, Schultz JB, Gulbins E, Weller M. Crm-A, bcl-2 and NDGA inhibit CD95L-induced apoptosis of malignant glioma cells at the level of caspase 8 processing. *Cell Death Differ.* 1998;5(10):894-900.

79. Peterson JD, Herzenberg LA, Vasquez K, Waltenbaugh C. Glutathione levels in antigen-presenting cells modulate Th1 and Th2 response patterns. *Proc Natl Acad Sci.* 1998;95(6):3071-3076.

80. Herzenberg LA, De Rosa SC, Dubs JG, Roederer M, Anderson MT, Ela SW, Deresinski SC, Herzenberg LA. Glutathione deficiency is associated with impaired survival in HIV disease. *Proc Natl Acad Sci* U S A. 1997;94(5):1967-1972.

81. Droge W, Herzenberg LA, Herzenberg LA, inventors; The Board of Trustees of the Leland Stanford Junior University, assignee. Treatment of diseases associated with cysteine deficiency. US patent 5 607 974. March 4, 1997.

82. Herzenberg LA, DeRosa SC, Herzenberg LA, Roederer M, inventors; The Board of Trustees of the Leland Stanford Junior University, assignee. Glutathione deficiency as a prognosis for survival in AIDS. US patent 5 843 785. December 1, 1998.

83. Talley AK, Dewhurst S, Perry SW, Dollard SC, Gummuluru S, Fine SM, New D, Epstein LG, Gendelman HE, Gelbard HA. Tumor necrosis factor alpha-induced apoptosis in human neuronal cells: protection by the antioxidant N-acetylcysteine and the genes bcl-2 and crmA. *Mol Cell Biol.* 1995;15(5):2359-2366.

Neurological Dysfunction in Chronic Fatigue Syndrome

Abhijit Chaudhuri, DM, MD, MRCP
Peter O. Behan, DSc, MD, FACP, FRCP

SUMMARY. Chronic fatigue syndrome (CFS), popularly known in Europe as myalgic encephalomyelitis (ME), is a common but not a new illness. CFS/ME was classified as a neurological disease by the World Health Organisation in 1993. Neurological dysfunction is considered the principal mechanism of both physical and mental fatigue in this condition. This article reviews the neurological symptoms of the epidemic and sporadic forms of the illness. Paroxysmal changes in the severity of symptoms (fatigue and neuropsychiatric) are the hallmark features in the natural history of this disease. Ion channel abnormality leading to neuronal instability in selective anatomical pathways (basal ganglia circuitry) is proposed as the possible mechanism of fluctuating fatigue and related symptoms in CFS. *[Article copies available for a fee from The Haworth Document Delivery Service: 1-800-342-9678. E-mail address: <getinfo@ haworthpressinc.com> Website: <http://www.haworthpressinc.com>]*

KEYWORDS. Ion channels, myalgic encephalomyelitis, basal ganglia

INTRODUCTION

Chronic fatigue syndrome (CFS) is a common disorder, occurring worldwide. It is however, not a new illness and had probably existed

Abhijit Chaudhuri is Clinical Lecturer in Neurology and Peter O. Behan is Professor of Neurology (Retired), University Department of Neurology, Institute of Neurological Sciences, Southern General Hospital, Glasgow G51 4TF, United Kingdom.
Address correspondence to: Abhijit Chaudhuri (E-mail: ac54p@udcf.gla.ac.uk).

[Haworth co-indexing entry note]: "Neurological Dysfunction in Chronic Fatigue Syndrome." Chaudhuri, Abhijit, and Peter O. Behan. Co-published simultaneously in *Journal of Chronic Fatigue Syndrome* (The Haworth Medical Press, an imprint of The Haworth Press, Inc.) Vol. 6, No. 3/4, 2000, pp. 51-68; and: *Chronic Fatigue Syndrome: Critical Reviews and Clinical Advances* (ed: Kenny De Meirleir, and Roberto Patarca-Montero) The Haworth Medical Press, an imprint of The Haworth Press, Inc., 2000, pp. 51-68. Single or multiple copies of this article are available for a fee from The Haworth Document Delivery Service [1-800-342-9678, 9:00 a.m. - 5:00 p.m. (EST). E-mail address: getinfo@haworthpressinc.com].

in the papyrus Ebers (circa 1400 BC) (1). Early cases of this syndrome were only recorded during epidemic outbreaks. The first epidemic of CFS to strike the Western civilisation dates back to the time of Henry VIII in England when one of his wives, Anne Boleyn, fell ill during an attack of what was called the "English Sweats" (2). In the nineteenth century, neurasthenia was the popular name for this illness, introduced by a New York neurologist, George Beard (3). In the middle of the twentieth century, neuromyasthenia replaced neurasthenia as the preferred term to take into account the muscle fatigue (myasthenia) that was an important symptom of this syndrome. Sporadic, pre-epidemic and epidemic forms of neurasthenia were already recognised in the late nineteenth century though it was the epidemic form that was most common (4). The geographic location where an epidemic had occurred provided names (e.g., Akureyri disease or Royal Free Hospital Disease); in addition, the names often reflected the suspected pathology of the illness (e.g., atypical poliomyelitis or poliomyelitis-like disease, myalgic encephalomyelitis). It is the sporadic form of the disease that is commonly encountered in present clinical practice.

Neurological symptoms and subtle neurological signs are well recognised in both the epidemic and sporadic forms of CFS (5). Neurological signs in some of the well studied epidemic outbreaks were, however, more dramatic. Another characteristic distinguishing feature of the epidemic outbreaks was the rapid evolution of neurological symptoms within the first week of the illness, often simulating poliomyelitis (6-8). We shall therefore discuss the neurological dysfunction in the epidemic and sporadic forms of CFS separately.

EPIDEMIC FORM

Typically, the epidemic forms got underway in the early summer or late autumn, a period when infections are common. All age groups may be affected; however, few cases were seen under 12 years of age. Observation suggested spread by personal contact or by droplet infection. High attack rate was consistently noted among nurses and ancillary institutional personnel, an observation that may be valid also in sporadic cases (9). Infection, either respiratory, diarrhoeal or meningitic, was the presumed cause for epidemic neuromyasthenia and the incubation period was calculated to be 5-7 days (10). Women outnumbered men and cardinal manifestations clearly pointed to the involvement of nervous, muscular, and reticuloendothelial system. Fatigue and lassitude were the hallmarks. Fever and lymphadenopathy were present in a number of cases with the onset of symptoms, supporting an infective aetiology.

Headache and dizziness appeared first; soon a myasthenic-like muscle dysfunction was noted in all where repetitive muscle contraction produced countenances of temporary weakness. This delay in muscle impulse generation was considered to be cerebral rather than myoneural. Symptoms of aseptic meningitis (photophobia, headache and normal cerebrospinal fluid) were seen in some, and a few patients had more severe symptoms suggestive of an encephalomyelitis with cranial nerve disturbances (ocular and facial palsies), diplopia, nystagmus, myoclonus, palatal paralysis and extensor plantar responses. Occasional cases appeared encephalopathic, called "benign subacute encephalitis" by Jelinek (11). This encephalopathy in the epidemic and sporadic disease was suspected to be toxic by workers like Shelokov who considered enteric bacteria as a source of the neurotoxin (12).

Neuropsychiatric symptoms were always present. These consisted of slowness of thinking, speaking and reading; anxiety was very common. Concentration and visual attention were impaired; patients complained that one sentence must be read and reread before it could be registered. Recent memory was defective, calculation at times impossible and patients were unable to attend to conversations or follow simple spoken instructions. Patients frequently experienced restlessness and insomnia at night and lethargy and somnolence during the day. The reversal of sleep rhythm was most severe during the first month. Other psychiatric symptoms included disinhibited behavior (emotional lability), weeping, irritability, apprehension, depression and neurosis. Interestingly, many of these symptoms, including weeping, occurred paroxysmally and were considered to be predominantly organic in origin.

In the cranial nerves, olfactory abnormalities have never been recorded. Blurred vision, diplopia and tiredness on reading were common complaints. Both pain and paresthesia were reported in the trigeminal distribution. Nonatrophic, transient facial weaknesses were seen. The auditory-vestibular nerve was probably the most frequently affected nerve. Vertigo and dizziness were early symptoms. A clinical picture with vertigo of sudden onset, usually accompanied by nausea, vomiting and followed by symptoms of lassitude and fatigue was described with infective epidemics dominated by gastrointestinal or respiratory infections (13). Vertigo and incoordination led to loss of balance in stance and gait. Painful dysphagia and heaviness of tongue ("glossoplegia") were also mentioned.

In the sensory system, pain was common and usually appeared in the second week, occurring in the muscles of the shoulder cap, neck, upper arm, back or extremities. The pain was transient and migratory. But at times, both pain and muscle spasm was severe enough to render muscles inactive, seemingly paralysed. Hyperpathia and hyperalgesia were common. Fog suggested "vegetative neuritis" as the name for this neurological syndrome (cited by Holt, 1965 [5]) to emphasise the frequent affection of the autonomic nervous system. Symptoms included vasomotor instability, angiospasm and secondary instability of body temperature with intolerance to heat and cold.

Movement disorders were not uncommon in the epidemic forms of the disease. Tremor was common and one epidemic was known by the descriptive term, encephalitis tremens (14). Chorea or choreiform movements were recorded to last as long as one year. Cogwheel rigidity was observed as well. Other movement disorders recorded in the literature include myoclonus, myokymia or fasciculations, torsion dystonia, and involuntary jerking. Hyperkinetic movements at the beginning was often followed by bradykinesia or lost motion, again to be replaced by hyperkinesia before resolution.

Provocative reports from the laboratory tests of epidemic neuromyasthenia linking its association with an infective agent were claimed (15) but whether the symptoms were the manifestation of a neurological infection remained unproven. Although the possibility that epidemic neuromyasthenia was a mass hysteria or psychoneurosis was espoused, this was dismissed by most investigators and physicians other than the psychiatrists.

Morbidity was significant, relapses were characteristic and for several weeks or months, the recovery period of most patients was characterised by fatigue, emotional lability, with slow gradual recovery. Chronic relapsing course was associated with exertion, inclement weather, menstruation in women and stresses. Disuse atrophy of muscles was rarely observed. As relapses recurred, apprehension, depression, anxiety and hostility complicated patient's illness. Death was extremely uncommon and when it occurred, it was months after the onset of symptoms and unrelated to neuromyasthenia. Pathological observations were inadequate but were reported to show non-specific, haemorrhagic congestion of the cortex and meninges. The lesions producing neural signs have never been demonstrated. However, neurons of the deep subcortical areas, spinal cord and autonomic nervous system were empirically implicated on clinical grounds.

In summary, epidemic neuromyasthenia had a distinctive clinical picture consisting of "headache, myalgia, myasthenia, encephalopathy, lymphadenopathy, relapse, morbidity and survivance" (5). It was; however, not strictly a monophasic illness since six years after the Akureyri outbreak, clinical findings in survivors showed persistence of fatigue, muscle pain, nervousness and disturbances of skin sensitivity (16), symptoms that are commonly present in patients with the current diagnosis of CFS acquired sporadically.

SPORADIC FORM

The sporadic cases differ in the severity of their neurological symptoms from the epidemic group. Neurological examination in these patients are more often normal. Only partly this difference may be related to the fact that patients are diagnosed at least six months after the onset of their symptoms to fulfill the current case definition of CFS (17). Like the epidemic form, more women than men are affected with sporadic CFS (18). The onset may be acute in upto one-third, occurring over hours to days but more subacute or insidious in the rest. Preceding infections, commonly viral, may be seen upto 80% of patients, often during a period of severe physical or mental stress (18). Only a minority of cases report no clear cut precipitating events. However, compared to the epidemic forms, sporadic CFS has less favourable prognosis (19).

Fatigue is indeed, the most important and central symptom of CFS. The fatigue is not only physical but also mental. Typically, there is significant post-exertional worsening of fatigue lasting for more than 24 hours and continuing for 48-72 hours, even upto 7 days. The type of fatigue exhibited by patients with CFS is different from the peripheral neuromuscular type of fatigue; on the other hand, fatigue symptoms in CFS patients are very similar to that seen in patients with MS or Parkinsonian disorders (20). We have termed this type of fatigue in chronic neurological disorders as "central fatigue" that is characterised by the presence of both physical and mental fatigue unlike the fatigue of peripheral neuromuscular disorders (e.g., myasthenia gravis or metabolic myopathies) where mental fatigue is either absent or seldom conspicuous. Although it is intuitive to assume that the mechanism of physical and mental fatigue that together constitute "central fatigue" in CFS must be same and come from the central nervous system, a peripheral contribution to the physical fatigue in CFS has never been satisfactorily excluded, especially in post-exertional fatigue lasting longer than 24 hours. Additionally, an early neurophysiological study in CFS patients had found increased jitter in single fibre electromyography (SFEMG) suggestive of abnormal neuromuscular conduction (21) that could not be later reduplicated. In this respect, physical fatigue in CFS was considered similar to the fatigue in post-polio syndrome (PPS) where increased jitter in SFEMG is demonstrable (22) and both peripheral (22) and central (23) role in post-polio fatigue symptoms have been speculated.

Physical fatigue: That the physical fatigue in CFS is exclusively or predominantly central is primarily supported by four sets of observations (24-28). First, CFS patients have delayed central motor conduction similar to that seen in MS patients (24). Second, there is delayed post-exercise facilitation of motor evoked potentials in CFS (25). Third, inability of CFS patients to fully activate skeletal muscles during intense, sustained exercise despite normal muscle membrane function, excitation-contraction coupling, intracellular and systemic metabolism (26). Fourthly, lack of sufficient histological evidence of skeletal muscle injury (27) or dysfunction (28) in the muscle biopsies of CFS patients.

Peripheral role in sustaining the physical component of fatigue in CFS or prolonging the post-exertional fatigue, first suspected from the observation of increased jitter in SFEMG (21), was supported by the evidence of abnormal oxidative metabolism of muscles (29) further confirmed by the phosphorus nuclear magnetic resonance spectroscopy (30,31) and finally, by the recent demonstration of mild aerobic defects in the cultured (*in vitro*) myoblasts from the skeletal muscles of CFS patients (32).

In a recently published article (33), 10 CFS patients and 10 control subjects were studied by an isometric fatiguing exercise test. During the exercise period, the maximum voluntary contractions (MVC) of the quadriceps were significantly higher in patients than in controls but both groups showed a parallel decline in force in keeping with a similar endurance capacity. Recovery was prolonged in the patient group but in addition, CFS patients showed a reduced MVC initially during the recovery after exercise and also at 24 hours unlike the control group who achieved initial MVCs during recovery comparable to the exercise period. This observation clearly suggests that CFS patients may have a centrally dependent "fatigue at rest" to account for the baseline difference of MVC before exercise; a similar endurance capacity in patients and controls during exercise would exclude any oxidative defect in muscles. However, the difference in the initial MVCs at the recovery phase and at 24 hours may be interpreted to suggest a defective peripheral mechanism related to "recharging" the muscle (resynthesis of the substrate and energy molecules, i.e., glycogen and ATP). However, decreased post-exercise facilitation of the motor evoked potentials in CFS on the other hand would suggest reduced post-exercise cortical excitability (25) and a central cause for post-exertional malaise. Another evidence that supports a central role (depressed cortical excitability) in post-exertional fatigue comes from the study of cognitive performance of CFS patients after exercise. As compared with healthy individuals, CFS subjects demonstrated impaired cognitive processing immediately and 24-hours after an exhaustive treadmill exercise although no differences were seen in the pre-exercise cognitive tests between the patients and healthy controls (34).

Thus, present data clearly point to a dominant central mechanism in the symptom of physical fatigue in CFS, both at rest and after exertion. Nevertheless, is it possible to reconcile the divergent views regarding the causation of physical fatigue in CFS (central vs. peripheral)? One explanation is that a basic metabolic or cellular defect that is variably expressed in the excitable tissues (nerves and muscles) can possibly account for this difference. Dysfunctional ion channels or disorders of mitochondrial respiration in CFS may, indeed, provide such a basis.

Mental fatigue: The neuropsychiatric symptoms in sporadic CFS are broadly similar to those seen during the epidemics though again, symptoms are slow in evolution and commonly less dramatic. The spectrum of the reported cognitive deficits include anomia, short-term memory and concentration difficulties. The degree of symptomatology may vary, but at its most severe form, CFS patients may be forced to abandon all intellectual pursuits and children with CFS discontinue schooling. Indeed, CFS is considered to be one of the commonest reasons for long-term sickness absence from school in UK (35). Some patients with CFS develop hypergraphia, i.e., keeping the most detailed records and long descriptions of all their symptoms and come to the clinic with interminable notes. Functional neuroimaging studies with PET (36) and SPECT (37,38) scans were abnormal both in children and in adults with CFS although the perfusion abnormalities were not specific or unifocal (39).

In our experience, anomia, reduced attention span (for both verbal and visual tasks), and concentration difficulties constitute the triad of cognitive dysfunction in CFS. These symptoms are always worse during and after any sustained physical and emotional stress. CFS patients are slower in psychomotor tasks, have impaired attention, slower retrieval from semantic memory, slow logical reasoning and show increased visual sensitivity (40). Interestingly, CFS patients with no concurrent psychopathology often have the greatest degree of neuropsychiatric impairment (41).

In a recently concluded trial of a large cohort of CFS patients, as compared to the age matched controls, baseline cognitive performance testing showed clearly impaired concentration, significantly slower speed of memory with preserved quality of memory. Significant prolongations of the N2 and P3 components with prolonged reaction time was found in the endogenous potential study of CFS patients (42). In another study, selective impairment of the auditory-task processing relative to the visually processed task was noticed in CFS patients when compared to patients with multiple sclerosis and controls (43).

Some workers consider the cognitive impairment in CFS supportive of a diffuse encephalopathic process of metabolic origin (41). There may be a correlation between the white matter abnormalities in the MRI brain scan and functional impairment in CFS (BH Natelson, personal communication). There is also evidence that hormones and neurotransmitters may play a role since in women with CFS, there is striking exacerbation of not only physical, but also mental symptoms during the menstrual phase. Women "whose menstrual phase had not been previously marked by hyper-irritability and emotional tension complained that they could not control themselves and flew into rages at what they realised were really insignificant frustrations and annoyances" (44).

Sleep: Unrefreshing sleep is a characteristic symptom in an average patient with CFS. At the beginning of the syndrome, patients are more often hypersomnolent and sleep for prolonged periods both during the day and night. Subsequently, these patients develop altered sleep rhythm with frequent, short periods of sleepiness during day time and have poor night time sleep. CFS patients also experience difficulty in falling asleep with broken sleep pattern and vivid dreams. Disordered sleep pattern, however, is not the cause of fatigue in CFS. Significant abnormalities in the polysomnographic studies of CFS patients are seldom seen (45). In one study, the quality of rapid-eye-movement (REM) sleep was similar in CFS and healthy controls (46). However, CFS patients have higher levels of sleep disruption, by both brief and longer awakenings. The mechanism of sleep disorder in CFS is not properly understood but possible explanations include (i) hypothalamic disorder causing circadian dysrhythmia and (ii) imbalance of neurotransmitters, especially affecting acetylcholine and/or serotonin.

Cranial nerves: Although an abnormality of the olfactory-limbic pathway is postulated in patients with multiple chemical sensitivities (47) (often sharing similar symptoms with CFS), olfactory symptoms are not reported by CFS patients. Visual symptoms, however, are relatively common. These include oscillopsia, photophobia and migrainous visual scotoma or temporary visual obscurations. In a study of patients with chronic primary fibromyalgia combined with dysesthesia, abnormal smooth pursuit and saccadic movements were documented in a high proportion of patients as opposed to controls, suggestive of subtle brain stem dysfunction (48). Perioral paresthesia and hemifacial sensory symptoms are less frequently reported (see below).

Vertigo is common and acute episodes in a CFS patient may last for a week to 10 days on average. Some CFS patients suffer from frequent spells of vertigo with gait disorder and dysequilibrium as the major physical symptom besides fatigue, similar to the sufferers of epidemic vertigo ("Pedersen's syndrome" [13]). A study of the vestibular function test demonstrated several abnormalities in CFS patients. They had poor performance in dynamic posturography, with greater number of falls and a reduction in the earth-vertical-axis (EVA) rotation gain. The CFS group, in addition, had abnormal optokinetic nystagmus during the course of the test. These results were interpreted to be more suggestive of central rather than peripheral vestibular dysfunction (49).

Motor symptoms: Short episodes of unexplained weakness affecting both legs, an arm or one side of body are described by some CFS patients who, on examination, very seldom show any evidence of

persistent motor weakness. Myokymia or benign muscle fasciculations are often reported in the early phase of the illness. Muscle stretch
reflexes are always preserved and are usually brisk. Unlike some of
the epidemic cases, plantar responses are invariably flexor in CFS.
Postural hand tremors are common and occasional patients may appear Parkinsonian. Rarely, myoclonus may be a symptom, probably as
a result of the supersensitive or hyperactive serotoninergic (5HT1A)
receptors in the brain stem and the spinal cord.

Gait kinetic studies at slow walking speed and short periods of
running in CFS patients had revealed a number of defects as compared
to the sedentary controls. Run time was significantly slower in CFS
patients who also had a smaller ratio of stride length divided by leg
length and smaller knee flexion during stance and swing phases than
controls (50). Another recent study confirmed the alteration of spatial-
temporal parameters of gait in CFS patients (51). Interestingly, abnormalities were present from the beginning of the gait, which indicated
that they were unlikely to be caused by the rapid increasing fatigue.
This observation further strengthens the notion of a direct involvement
of the central nervous system in CFS.

Sensory symptoms: These are extremely common. Both diffuse
muscle aches and pain as well as fibromyalgia are frequently reported.
New-onset daily headache, often migraine-type, is another common
symptom. Persistent or paroxysmal hemi-paresthesia, altered acral
perception of thermal sensations (at times with reversal of cold and
hot) and symptoms very similar to migratory neuropathy can be seen
in CFS patients. Patients with ciguatera fish poisoning display symptoms of fatigue, perioral paresthesia and altered thermal sensibility
identical to those reported by CFS patients (52). Ciguatera toxin,
however, is a sodium channel inactivator (53) and some of the sensory
symptoms in these patients are considered to be due to the sodium
channel blockade in the nerves (52).

Autonomic symptoms: Vagal afferent tone was found to be reduced
during paced breathing in CFS patients (54). Abnormal response to
upright table tilt testing was frequently observed in a study (55). This
phenomenon, called neurally mediated hypotension, led to the development of severe presyncope with warmth, light-headedness, nausea
and sweating in the tested CFS patients. Other symptoms of dysauto-
nomia in CFS patients include orthostatic changes in blood pressure
(10-20 mm Hg), paroxysms of sweating especially at night, abnormal

colonic motility (similar to irritable bowel syndrome), increased frequency of urination, erectile dysfunction in men and dysparuenia in women. A sympathetic overactivity was observed in CFS patients when they were exposed to stress (56).

Alcohol intolerance: Alcohol intolerance, leading to an early "blackout" or a next day severe hangover is common in CFS patients many of whom are forced to abandon their social drinking. Although the mechanism of alcohol intolerance in CFS patients has not been understood, serotonin supersensitivity may be a likely explanation since it has been proposed that alcoholic blackouts result from a disorder of central serotoninergic neurotransmission. Plasma levels of the serotonin precursor, tryptophan, are decreased in male alcoholics with history of blackouts due to ethanol intoxication (57) and a trial of serotonin reuptake inhibitor zimelidine had shown improvement in memory function in moderately intoxicated subjects (58).

Neuroendocrine changes: Abnormalities of neurohypophyseal function has always been suspected in CFS patients. Indeed, abnormal water excretion, idiopathic cyclic oedema, sleep disorder, irregular menstrual cycles, fluctuations in weight and autonomic symptoms in CFS patients led to an extensive evaluation of multiple neuroendocrine axes and testing for the anterior and posterior pituitary functions. These showed a variable subsensitivity of CFS patients to vasopressin, supersensitivity to serotonin (and possibly to acetylcholine and dopamine) but most consistently, a hypoactive hypothalamic-pituitary-adrenal (HPA) axis (18). This hypoactive HPA axis is considered the basis for poor stress response ("cowering response") in CFS patients and is also responsible for the generation of pro-inflammatory cytokines that may exacerbate symptoms like asthma (59). Chocolate craving is another interesting symptom seen in approximately a third of all CFS patients (usually women) some of whom also report mood changes dependent on day-light exposure similar to the patients with seasonal affective disorder, a condition caused by low serotonin levels (60).

In summary, the neurological symptoms of chronic fatigue syndrome appear to be multifocal, almost exclusively central and autonomic with some peripheral features. These symptoms are not uniform and in a given case, all the symptoms, including fatigue, may fluctuate in their severity. This variability of symptoms in CFS forms the basis of the experience of "good days" and "bad days" reported by an average patient. The fluctuation of symptoms, including fatigue, is the hallmark of CFS.

THE MECHANISM OF NEUROLOGICAL DYSFUNCTION

It is difficult, in the confines of the established disease models, to offer a simplistic explanation for the neurological dysfunction seen in patients with the epidemic and the more common, sporadic form of CFS. A dysfunctional ion channel affecting neurotransmitter release or cytokine function is one of the possible explanations (61). However, it is also important to identify the neuroanatomic pathways where dysfunctional ion channels are operative.

The anatomy of chronic fatigue: In many ways, post-polio syndrome (PPS) of fatigue still remains an useful paradigm to explore the mechanism of fatigue in CFS.The neuropathology and research in this area have clearly pointed to a central role of fatigue that has been supported by a recently failed trial of pyridostigmine in improving the symptom of fatigue in PPS despite the fact that peripheral neuromuscular conduction had improved in treated patients (as measured by jitter in SFEMG) (62). Post-mortem examination performed 50 years ago showed selective damage to the midbrain reticular formation, substantia nigra, thalamic, hypothalamic and caudate nuclei, putamen, globus pallidus and locus ceruleus caused by poliovirus infection (63). Role of basal ganglia in fatigue mechanism is also supported by the observation of fatigue in patients with idiopathic Parkinson's disease (PD) that is characterised by the loss of melanin-containing neurones in the substantia nigra pars compacta. Fatigue in PD is extremely common and is often considered a "warning sign" of oncoming PD since it may antedate the development of motor symptoms by several months. Patients symptomatic of the Parkinsonian triad (rigidity, bradykinesia and tremor) demonstrate rapid fatiguability of motor tasks (64).

We believe that basal ganglia pathways are involved in the mechanism of the chronic fatigue symptoms that comprise of both physical and mental fatigue. This is not identical with the brain-fatigue generator model in PPS proposed by Bruno et al. (65) but shares the similar view that the central fatigue is due to a failure of normal cortical and brainstem activation process. Given the complexity of the basal ganglia circuitry and neurotransmission, it would be naive to suggest that a single neurotransmitter abnormality or loss of a single projection system in the basal ganglia would be responsible for *central fatigue* (comprising symptoms of both physical and mental fatigue).

The interaction between ion channels, neurotransmitters and specific neuroanatomical network: Paroxysmal disorders like idiopathic epilepsy and common migraine provide important models for CFS where fatigue symptoms fluctuate on a day to day basis. In common migraine, paroxyms of headache are produced by an interaction between altered ion channel (calcium) excitability and neurotransmitter (serotonin) sensitivity acting on a specific anatomic pathway (trigeminovasscular and hypothalamic). In idiopathic epilepsy, both voltage-gated (potassium and sodium) and ligand-gated (nicotinic acetylcholine and NMDA-subtype) ion channels are considered responsible; the neurotransmitters involved are either an excess of glutamate (excitotoxic) or deficiency of GABA (inhibitory). The neuranatomic pathways are cortical foci, thalamus and cortical projection system to the other brain areas and the reticular activating system.

We propose that a similar model of pathogenic mechanism is responsible for the symptoms in epidemic neuromyasthenia, myalgic encephalomyelitis and the sporadic form of the same illness currently known as CFS. Throughout this review, we have emphasised the nature of *paroxysmal* changes in the severity of symptoms, both physical and mental fatigue and the neuropsychiatric changes, that were well recognised in the epidemic outbreaks of the illness (5) and are commonly experienced in the sporadic form (61) of CFS. Based on our previous work, we suspected potassium ion channels to be the key players and the alteration of the neuronal excitability caused by potassium channelopathy as the basis of the fluctuating nature of CFS symptoms (61). An ion channel dysfunction in CFS will also explain the phenomenon of increased jitter in SFEMG that was postulated to be due to the abnormal muscle membrane function in the original study (21). We, however, acknowledge the role of basal ganglia as the neural integrator for the motor and motivational aspects of higher cortical and limbic activities (66) and we believe that a failure of this function, induced by an interaction between the ion channels and neurotransmitters, will cause CFS while the fluctuations in the symptom severity are caused by ion channelopathy altering the neurotransmitter signals to the excitable tissues. The neurotransmitters that are directly involved are serotonin, dopamine and acetylcholine or more appropriately, a balance between these three neurotransmitters within the basal ganglia network. The final result is a shift in the neuronal excitability of the cortical, limbic and brainstem areas giving rise to the characteristic constellation of symptoms seen in CFS. Downregulation of the hypothalamic-piltuitary-adrenal (HPA) axis in CFS is probably a secondary phenomenon and an adaptive response to the changes in the neurotransmitter system rather than the primary event responsible for the fatigue symptoms. Immunological dysfunction and aberrant cytokine responses in CFS (18) are likely to be the consequences of this alteration in the HPA axis (59).

CONCLUSION

The anatomical pathways and the chemical substrate for fatigue in the disorders of central nervous system are not fully understood. There is extensive, bidirectional linkage between the basal ganglia and cerebral cortex that includes several functional and anatomically distinct circuits regulating motor activity and more complex cognitive bahaviours. Basal ganglia are involved in the higher order, cognitive aspects of motor control and these neurons also influence many other functions through their extensive connections with the association cortex, hypothalamus and limbic structures (66).

Alteration in the normal flow of sequential activation within the basal ganglia system affecting the neural integrator will cause *central fatigue*. This would probably the result of a combination of events that may include structural damage to basal ganglia (e.g., in encephalitis lethargica), ion channel dysfunction (chronic ciguatera poisoning) or altered neurotransmitter balance (Parkinson's disease), acting either singly or in combination. Central-type fatigue may occur transiently in the setting of an inherited ion channel disease (channelopathy), as in paroxysmal dyskinesias and more persistently, in acquired neurodegenerative diseases like PD.

In this paper, we are proposing a complex interaction between ion channels, neurotransmitters and specific neuroanatomic areas in the brain to be responsible for *central fatigue* in CFS comprising the symptoms of both physical and mental fatigue. This is not a new model since comparable mechanisms of pathogenesis are currently accepted for common migraine and idiopathic epilepsy, the latter thought to be a psychiatric illness until the second half of the twentieth century. A better understanding of the anatomy and neurotransmission of the basal ganglia pathways would be extremely important in the therapeutic management of *central fatigue*. Unravelling the neurobiology of basal ganglia and their interaction with ion channels and neurotransmitters integrating motivation, motor and emotional activities will have important connotation not only in the treatment of CFS but also in PD, PPS and MS.

REFERENCES

1. The Papyrus Ebers: the greatest Egyptian medical document. Translated by B. Ebbell. Copenhagen, Levin & Munksgaard 1937; 108-13.

2. Sylvest E. Epidemic myalgia: Bornholm disease. London, Oxford University Press, 1934.

3. Beard G. Neurasthenia, or nervous exhaustion. Bost Med Sur J 1869; 3: 217-221.

4. Ramsay A. Epidemic neuromyasthenia: 1955-1978. Postgrad Med J 1978; 54: 718-21.

5. Holt GW. Epidemic neuromyasthenia: the sporadic form. Am J Med Sci 1965; 249: 98-112.

6. Ramsay AM, O'Sullivan E. Encephalomyelitis simulating poliomyelitis. Lancet 1956; 1: 761-64.

7. Sumner DW. Further outbreak of a disease resembling poliomyelitis. Lancet 1956; 1: 764-66.

8. Ramsay AM. Encephalomyelitis in North West London. A disease simulating poliomyelitis and hysteria. Lancet 1957; 2: 1196-1200.

9. Jason LA, Wagner L, Rosenthal S, et al. Estimating the prevalence of chronic fatigue syndrome among nurses. Am J Med 1998; 105(3A): 91S-93S.

10. Acheson ED. The clinical syndrome variously called benign myalgic encephalomyelitis, Icelandic disease and epidemic neuromyasthenia. Am J Med 1959; 26: 569-95.

11. Jellinek JE. Benign encephalomyelitis. Lancet 1956; 2: 494-95.

12. Shelokov A, Habel K, Verder E, Welsh W. Epidemic neuromyasthenia: An outbreak of poliomyelitis-like illness in student nurses. N Engl J Med 1957; 257: 345-55.

13. Pedersen E. Epidemic vertigo. Brain 1959; 82: 566-80.

14. Wright J, Morley DC. Encephalitis tremens. Lancet 1958; 1: 871-73.

15. Pellew RAA, Miles JAR. Further investigations on a disease resembling poliomyelitis seen in Adelaide. Med J Aust 1955; 42: 480-82.

16. Sigurdsson B, Gudmundsson KR. Clinical findings six years after the outbreak of Akureyri disease. Lancet 1956; 1: 766-67.

17. Fukuda K, Strauss SE, Hickie I, et al. The chronic fatigue syndrome: a comprehensive approach to case definition and study. Ann Intern Med 1994; 121: 953-59.

18. Chaudhuri A, Behan WMH, Behan PO. Chronic fatigue syndrome. Proc R Coll Physicians Edinb 1998; 28: 150-63.

19. Levine PH, Snow PG, Ranum BA, Paul C, Holmes MJ. Epidemic neuromyasthenia and chronic fatigue syndrome in West Otago, New Zealand. A 10-year follow up. Arch Int Med 1997; 157: 750-4.

20. Chaudhuri A, Behan PO. Overlap syndromes of chronic fatigue. CNS 1(2): 16-20.

21. Jamal GA, Hansen S. Electrophysiological studies in the post-viral fatigue syndrome. J Neurol Neurosurg & Psychiat 1985; 48: 691-4.

22. Trojan DA, Gendron D, Cashman NR. Anticholinesterase-responsive neuromuscular junction transmission defects in post-poliomyelitis fatigue. J Neurol Sci 1993; 114: 170-77.

23. Bruno RL, Sapolsky R, Zimmerman JR, Frick NM. The pathophysiology of a central cause of post-polio fatigue. Ann NY Acad Sci 1995; 753: 257-75.

24. Hilgers A, Frank J, Bolte P. Prolongation of central motor conduction time in chronic fatigue syndrome. J Chronic Fatigue Synd 1998; 4(2): 23-32.

25. Samii A, Wassermann EM, Ikoma K et al. Decreased post-exercise facilitation of motor evoked potentials in patients with chronic fatigue syndrome or depression. Neurology 1996; 47(6): 1410-4.

26. Kent-Braun JA, Sharma KR, Weiner MW, Massie B, Miller RG. Central basis of muscle fatigue in chronic fatigue syndrome. Neurology 1993; 43: 125-31.

27. Behan PO, Behan WHM, Bell EJ. The postviral fatigue syndrome–an analysis of findings in 50 cases. J Infect 1985; 10: 211-22.

28. Lane RJ, Barrett MC, Woodrow D et al. Muscle fibre characteristics and lactate responses to exercise in chronic fatigue syndrome. J Neurol Neurosurg & Psychiat 1998; 64: 362-7.

29. McCully KK, Natelson BH, Iotti S, Sisto S, Leigh JS Jr. Reduced oxidative muscle metabolism in chronic fatigue syndrome. Muscle & Nerve 1996; 19: 621-5.

30. Barnes PRJ, Taylor DJ, Kemp GJ, Radda GK. Skeletal muscle bioenergetics in the chronic fatigue syndrome. J Neurol Neurosurg & Psychiat 1993; 56: 679-83.

31. Wong R, Lopaschuk G, Zhu G et al. Skeletal muscle metabolism in chronic fatigue syndrome. In vivo assessment by ^{31}P nuclear magnetic resonance spectroscopy. Chest 1992; 102: 1716-22.

32. Behan WMH, Holt J, Kay DH, Moonie P. In vitro study of muscle aerobic metabolism in chronic fatigue syndrome. J Chronic Fatigue Synd 1999; 5(1): 3-16.

33. Paul L, Wood L, Behan WMH, McLaren WM. Demonstration of delayed recovery from fatiguing exercise in chronic fatigue syndrome. European J Neurol 1999; 6: 63-9.

34. LaManca JJ, Sisto DA, De Luca J et al. Influence of exhaustive treadmill exercise on cognitive functioning in chronic fatigue syndrome. Am J Med 1998; 105(3A): 59S-65S.

35. Dowsett EG, Colby J. Long term sickness absence due to ME/CFS in UK schools: an epidemiological study with medical and educational implications. J Chronic Fatigue Synd 1997; 3: 29-42.

36. Tirelli U, Chierichetti F, Tavio M et al. Brain Positron Emission Tomography (PET) in chronic fatigue syndrome: preliminary data. Am J Med 1998; 105(3A): 54S-58S.

37. Patterson J, Aitchison F, Wyper DJ et al. SPECT brain imaging in chronic fatigue syndrome. EOS-J Immunol Immunopharmacol 1995; 15: 53-58.

38. Goldberg M, Meena I, Darcourt J. NeuroSPECT findings in children with chronic fatigue syndrome. Proceedings AACFS Conference 1994; 79.

39. Schwartz RB, Komaroff AL, Garada BM et al. SPECT imaging of the brain: comparison of findings in patients with chronic fatigue syndrome, AIDS dementia complex and major unipolar depression. AJR 1994; 162: 943-51.

40. Smith AP, Behan PO, Bell W, Millar K, Bakheit M. Behavioural problems associated with the chronic fatigue syndrome. Br J Psychology 1993; 84: 411-23.

41. Christodoulou C, DeLuca J, Lange G et al. Relation between neuropsychological impairment and functional disability in patients with chronic fatigue syndrome. J Neurol Neurosurg Psychiat 1998; 64: 431-4.

42. Prasher D, Smith A, Findley L. Sensory and cognitive-event related potentials in myalgic encephalomyelitis. J Neurol Neurosurg & Psychiat 1990; 53: 247-53.

43. Johnson SK, DeLuca J. Selective impairment of auditory processing in chronic fatigue syndrome: a comparison with multiple sclerosis and healthy controls. Perceptual and Motor Skills 1996; 83: 51-62.

44. Deisher JB. Benign myalgic encephalomyelitis (Iceland Disease) in Alaska. Northwest Medicine 1957; 56: 1451-56.

45. Sharpley A, Clemens A, Hawton K, Sharpe M. Do patients with "pure" chronic fatigue syndrome (neurasthenia) have abnormal sleep? Psychosomatic Medicine 1997; 59: 592-6.

46. Fischler B, LeBon O, Hoffman G et al. Sleep anomalies in the chronic fatigue syndrome. A comorbidity study. Neuropsychobiology 1997; 35: 115-22.

47. Bell IR, Miller CS, Schwartz GE. An olfactory-limbic model of multiple chemical sensitivity syndrome: possible relationship to kindling and affective spectrum disorders. Biol Psychiatry 1991; 32: 218-42.

48. Rosenhall U, Johansson G, Orndahl G. Eye motility dysfunction in chronic primary fibromyalgia with dysesthesia. Scand J Rehab Med 1987; 19: 139-45.

49. Ash-Bernal R, Wall II C, Komaroff AL et al. Vestibular function test anomalies in patients with chronic fatigue syndrome. Acta Otolaryngol 1995; 115: 9-17.

50. Boda WI, Natelson BH, Sisto SA, Tapp WN. Gait abnormalities in chronic fatigue syndrome. J Neurol Sci 1995; 131: 156-61.

51. Saggini R, Pizzigallo E, Vecchiet J, Macellari V, Giacomozzi C. Alteration of spatial-tempral parameters of gait in chronic fatigue syndrome patients. J Neurol Sci 1998; 154:18-25.

52. Cameron J, Capra MF. The basis of the paradoxic disturbance of temperature perception in ciguatera poisoning. J Toxicol 1993; 31: 571-79.

53. Bidard JN, Vijverberg HPM, Frelin C. Ciguatoxin is a novel type of Na+ channel toxin. J Biological Chemistry 1984; 259: 8353-57.

54. Sisto SA, Tapp W, Drastal S et al. Vagal tone is reduced during paced breathing in patients with the chronic fatigue syndrome. Clinical Autonomic Research 1995; 5: 139-43.

55. Bou-Holaigh I, Rowe PC, Kan JS, Calkins H. The relationship between neurally mediated hypotension and chronic fatigue syndrome. JAMA 1995; 274: 961-67.

56. De Becker P, Dendale P, De Meirleir K et al. Autonomic testing in patients with chronic fatigue syndrome. Am J Med 1998; 105(3A): 22S-26S.

57. Branchey L, Branchey M, Zucker D, Shaw S, Lieber CS. Association between low plasma tryptophan and blackouts in male alcoholic patients. Alcoholism (NY) 1985; 9: 393-5.

58. Weingartner H, Buchsbaum MS, Linnoila M. Zimelidine effects on memory impairments produced by ethanol. Life Sci 1983; 33: 2159-63.

59. McEwen BS. Protective and damaging effects of stress mediators. N Engl J Med 1998; 338: 171-79.

60. Terman M, Levine SM, Terman JS, Doherty S. Chronic fatigue syndrome and seasonal affective disorder: comorbidity, diagnostic overlap and implications for treatment. Am J Med 1998; 105(3A): 115S-124S.

61. Chaudhuri A, Behan PO. Chronic fatigue syndrome is an acquired neurological channelopathy. Hum Psychopharmacol Clin Exp 1999; 14: 7-17.

62. Trojan DA, Collet J-P, Shapiro S, et al. A multi-center, randomized, double-blinded trial of pyridostigmine in postpolio syndrome. Neurology 1999; 63: 1225-33.

63. Luthan JA. Epidemic poliomyelitis. Some pathological observations on human material. Arch Pathol 1946; 42: 245-60.

64. Adams RD, Victor M, Ropper AH. Principles of Neurology, sixth edition. New York, McGraw Hill 1998; pp 497-507.

65. Bruno RL, Frick NM, Creange SJ, et al. Polioencephalitis and the brain fatigue generator model of post-viral fatigue syndromes. J Chronic Fatigue Synd 1996; 2: 5-27.

66. Nauta HJW. The relationship of basal ganglia to the limbic system. In: Vinken PJ, Bruyn GW(eds). Handbook of Clinical Neurology, vol 49. Amsterdam, Elsevier Science, pp 19-32.

Immunology of Chronic Fatigue Syndrome

Roberto Patarca-Montero, MD, PhD
Timothy Mark, MD
Mary Ann Fletcher, PhD
Nancy G. Klimas, MD

SUMMARY. A review of the literature on the immunology of CFS reveals that people who have Chronic Fatigue Syndrome (CFS) have two basic problems with immune function that have been documented by most research groups: 1. immune activation, as demonstrated by elevation of activated T lymphocytes, including cytotoxic T cells, as well as elevations of circulating cytokines; and 2. poor cellular function, with low natural killer cell cytotoxicity (NKCC), poor lymphocyte response to mitogens in culture, and frequent immunoglobulin deficiencies, most often IgG1 and IgG3. These findings have a waxing and waning temporal pattern which is consistent with episodic immune dysfunction (with predominance of so called T-helper type 2 and proinflammatory cytokines and low NKCC and lymphoproliferation) that can be associated as cause or effect of the physiological and psychological function derangement and/or activation of latent viruses or other pathogens. The interplay of these factors can account for the perpetuation of disease with remission/exacerbation cycles. Therapeutic intervention aimed at induction of a more favorable cytokine expression pattern and immune status is discussed. *[Article copies available for a fee from The Haworth Document Delivery Service: 1-800-342-9678. E-mail address: <getinfo@haworthpressinc.com> Website: <http://www.haworthpressinc.com>]*

Roberto Patarca-Montero, Timothy Mark, Mary Ann Fletcher, and Nancy G. Klimas are affiliated with the E. M. Papper Laboratory of Clinical Immunology, Department of Medicine (R-42), University of Miami School of Medicine, P.O. Box 016960, Miami, FL 33101.

Address correspondence to: Roberto Patarca-Montero (E-mail: rpatarca@pol.net).

[Haworth co-indexing entry note]: "Immunology of Chronic Fatigue Syndrome." Patarca-Montero, Roberto et al. Co-published simultaneously in *Journal of Chronic Fatigue Syndrome* (The Haworth Medical Press, an imprint of The Haworth Press, Inc.) Vol. 6, No. 3/4, 2000, pp. 69-107; and: *Chronic Fatigue Syndrome: Critical Reviews and Clinical Advances* (ed: Kenny De Meirleir, and Roberto Patarca-Montero) The Haworth Medical Press, an imprint of The Haworth Press, Inc., 2000, pp. 69-107. Single or multiple copies of this article are available for a fee from The Haworth Document Delivery Service [1-800-342-9678, 9:00 a.m. - 5:00 p.m. (EST). E-mail address: getinfo@haworthpressinc.com].

KEYWORDS. T cells, immunoglobulins, cytokines, natural killer cells

INTRODUCTION

The nervous and immune systems respond to internal and external challenges and communicate and regulate each other by means of shared or system-unique hormones, growth factors, neurotransmitters and neuromodulators. Similar alterations in central catecholamine neurotransmitter levels are associated with immune activity and stressor exposure, alterations that are more pronounced in aged as opposed to younger animals (1). For example, a decreased norepinephrine turnover in the hypothalamus and brain stem of rats occurs at the peak of the immune response to sheep red blood cells (2,3), and increased serotonin metabolism is associated with depressed Arthus reaction and plaque-forming cell response in rats stressed either by overcrowding lasting two weeks or more or by repeated immunobilization for four days (4,5). The long-term effects of these acute changes are evidenced by chronic variable stress which facilitates tumor growth (6) and is associated with immune dysregulation in multiple sclerosis (7). The hypothalamic-pituitay-adrenal axis plays a pivotal role in stress-mediated changes, and stimulation of corticotropin-releasing factor in the central nervous system (8,9) has been shown to suppress rapidly a variety of immune responses, an effect which can be blocked by infusion into the brain of alpha-melanocyte-stimulating hormone, a tridecapeptide derived from pro-opiomelanocortin (10).

Besides external stimuli, intrinsic imbalances in neurotransmitter levels affect the immune system either directly by acting on immunocompetent cells or indirectly via induction of hormonal secretions. For instance, depression is associated with neurotransmitter imbalances and with decreased natural killer cell cytotoxic activity (11-14). Moreover, several studies have documented the existence of striking physiologic, neuroendocrine, metabolic, and pharmacologic differences between depressed and normal subjects and between depressed and severely ill subjects (15-20).

The examples mentioned above illustrate the fact that disorders, or persistent noxious stimulation, of the neuroimmunological circuitry can lead to, or result from, neurological, immunological, psychiatric or multiorgan pathology. The latter link has encouraged a search for

neuroimmunological markers with functional or pathological correlates.

Although the cause of CFS remains to be elucidated, many studies
summarized herein have provided evidence for abnormalities in immunological markers among individuals diagnosed with CFS. A clear
picture has not been achieved because of the noticeable variability in
the nature and magnitude of the findings reported by different groups
(21,22). Moreover, little support has been garnered for an association
between the latter abnormalities and the diverse physical and health
status changes in the CFS population. For instance, Buchwald and
coworkers (23) concluded that although a subset of CFS patients with
immune system activation can be identified, serum markers of inflammation and immune activation are of limited diagnostic useful-
ness in the evaluation of patients with CSF and chronic fatigue because changes in their values may reflect an intercurrent, transient,
common condition, such as an upper respiratory infection, or may be
the result of an ongoing illness-associated process. On the other hand,
Patarca and colleagues (24,25) have found that CFS patients can be
categorized based on immunological findings. It is also worth noting
that although the degree of overlap between distributions of soluble
immune mediators in CFS and controls has fueled criticism on the
validity or clinical significance of immune abnormalities in CFS, the
latter degree of overlap is not unique to CFS and is also present, for
instance, in sepsis syndrome and HIV-1-associated disease, clinical
entities where studies of immune abnormalities are providing insight
into pathophysiology (26).

The aim of this report is to comprehensively review the literature on
the immunology of CFS, to formulate consensus by majority conclusions when possible, and to discuss how this knowledge may contribute to the understanding of the physiological and psychological function changes seen in CFS. Immunological status findings will be
reviewed and discussed at three levels: immune cell phenotypic distributions, immune cell function, and cytokines and other soluble immune mediators.

IMMUNE CELL PHENOTYPIC DISTRIBUTIONS

Analysis of the complex interactions underlying immune responses
was greatly facilitated by the development of monoclonal antibodies

to various surface proteins on lymphoid cells, which defined functionally distinct subsets (27-29). Such analysis has also demonstrated that each type of lymphoid cell is genetically programmed to carry out defined immunological functions that are predictable on the basis of surface phenotype (29).

Surface-marker phenotyping of peripheral blood lymphoid cells has also allowed insight into the cellular basis of immune dysfunction associated with pathologies of the central nervous system with diverse causes, including viral, autoimmune, and genetic, among others (see, e.g., refs. 30-36). Several reports also documented alterations in the distribution of various lymphoid cell subsets among CFS patients. Certain discrepancies in the findings from different study groups can be attributed to group nonequivalences on diverse parameters such as demographic variables (gender, age, socioeconomic status), medical status variables predating onset of disease, medication use, concomitant substance abuse, nutritional status, and the effects of time of sample collection (diurnal or seasonal variations; 31,37-44).

T Lymphocytes

CD4+ T cells (helper-inducer cells) are the principal source of "help" for antibody production by B cells in response to T-cell-dependent antigenic stimulation, as well as inducers of cytotoxic and suppressor T-cell function (CD8+ cells; 28). Discrepant results have been reported in reference to CD4 and CD8 cell counts in CFS patients. Straus and colleagues (45) reported a statistically higher percentage of CD4+ lymphocytes with normal numbers of CD8+ cells and CD4/CD8 ratio; Jones (46) and colleagues (47,48), Borysiewicz et al. (49), Gupta and Vayuveguta (50), Landay (51), Lloyd (52) and Tirelli (53) and their coworkers found normal percentages of CD4+ and CD8+ cells as well as a normal CD4/CD8 ratio; Lloyd and coauthors (54) found decreased numbers of both CD4+ and CD8+ cells; Buchwald and Komaroff (55) found reduced numbers of CD8+ cells and higher-than-normal CD4/CD8 ratios; and Klimas and colleagues (56) found that most CFS subjects studied had a normal number of CD4+ cells and an elevated number of CD8+ cells that resulted in a decrease in the CD4/CD8 ratio (56). Decreased CD4/CD8 ratios in 2% to 100% of patients have been demonstrated by other investigators (46-49,57-59).

These conflicting results may be associated with the fluctuation in clinical manifestations of these patients or with other factors mentioned previously. In fact, several researchers have detected fluctuations in several immunological parameters and in the severity of symptoms in longitudinal follow-up investigations of patients with CFS. Moreover, Mawle and coworkers (60) found that although only marginal differences in cytokine responses and in cell surface markers were apparent in the total CFS population they studied, when the patients were subgrouped by type of disease onset (gradual or sudden) or by how well they were feeling on the day of testing, more pronounced differences were seen. It is also worth noting that although Peakman and coworkers did not find significant differences in the percentage levels of total CD3+, CD4+, CD8+, and activated, naive and memory T-cell subsets between CFS subjects and controls, they cryopreserved the cells before flow cytometric analysis and cryopreservation can differentially affect the representation of T-cell subsets (61).

A study by Sandman and colleagues (62) found that elevated CD4+ and CD8+ cell counts in CFS patients were related to decreases in priming of memory, speed of memory scanning and increases in errors on a memory fragility test. However the latter study did not control for depression severity, and it is not clear whether the finding is related to co-morbid depression or to CFS itself.

Klimas and co-workers (56) found a decreased proportion of CD4+CD45RA+ cells, which are associated with suppressor/cytotoxic cell induction (63) but Natelson and coworkers (64) found no significant change in the proportions of CD4+CD45RA+ and CD4+CD45RO+ cells in CFS patients. Franco and coinvestigators (65) also described a decrease in the number of CD4+CD45RA+ lymphocytes in two patients with severe, chronic, active Epstein-Barr virus (EBV) infection; one of the two patients showed a persistent diminished number of cells despite clinical improvement with interleukin-2 (IL-2) treatment. Several publications have associated alterations in the latter subset with a number of clinical entities, particularly autoimmune diseases (22,33, 63,66-68).

Increased numbers of T cells expressing the activation marker CD26, probably as a result of CD8+ activation, have also been reported in CFS patients (56). In this respect, an increased proportion of CD8+ cells expressing the activation marker human leukocyte antigen (HLA)-DR (51,56,69,70) have been reported in CFS patients, whereas normal proportions of CD4+ T cells co-expressing the HLA-DR marker or the IL-2 receptor (CD25) were found in one study (51), normal proportions of CD8+ CD38+, CD8+CD11b-, CD8+HLA-DR+ and CD8+CD28+ were found in another study (64), and normal proportions of CD8+HLA-DR+ and CD8+CD38+ were found by Swanink and coworkers (71). In contraposition to the latter findings, Hassan and colleagues (70) found significantly decreased expression of CD28 on CD8 cells and Barker (69), Landay (51) and Swanink (71) and their coworkers found significantly decreased expression of CD11b on CD8 cells. Higher expression of CD38 on CD8 cells was found by Barker (69), Landay (51) and Peakman (72) and their coworkers.

It is worth noting that relatively higher proportions of HLA-DR+ T cells have been reported in a number of autoimmune disorders (73-77), and that Hassan and coworkers (70) found that CFS patients with increased HLA-DR expression had significantly lower Short Form-36 health questionnaire (SF-36) total scores, worse body pains, and poorer general health perception and physical functioning scores. The increased expression of class II antigens and the reduced expression of the costimulatory receptor CD28, which is a marker of terminally differentiated cells, lend further support to the concept of immunoactivation of T-lymphocytes in CFS and may be consistent with the notion of a viral etiopathogenesis in the illness.

We studied the association between CFS physical symptoms, illness burden and lymphocyte activation markers in 27 newly-recruited CFS patients (78). Elevations in T-helper/inducer cells were associated with a greater frequency and severity of tender lymph nodes, greater severity of memory and concentration difficulties and headaches. Greater numbers of activated T cells (CD2+CD3+CD26+) were associated with a greater frequency of tender lymph nodes and cognitive difficulties while more activated cytotoxic/suppressor cells (CD8+CD38+HLA-DR+) were associated with greater severity of tender lymph nodes, fatigue and sleep problems. Conversely, lower percentages of regulatory cells such as CD3+CD8+ were associated with a greater number of cognitive difficulties, greater Sickness Impact profile(SIP)-Total, SIP Physical Impairment, and an increased frequency and severity of memory problems, increased frequency of headaches, and increased severity of fatigue. Thus, among CFS patients the degree of cellular immune activation is associated with the severity of CFS-related physical symptoms, cognitive complaints, and perceived illness burden.

B Lymphocytes

Gupta (50), Klimas (56), Landay (51), Lloyd (52) and Barker (69) and their colleagues found normal levels of CD20+ resting B cells, whereas other teams reported both increased and decreased levels (49,53,55,59). The proportion of CD5-bearing B cells was found to be increased in two studies (53,56) or decreased in one study (51). B cells bearing the cell marker CD5 have been associated with autoimmunity (79).

Natural Killer Cells

Klimas (56), Morrison (80), Peakman (72) and Tirelli (53) and their associates found increased numbers of NK cells, whereas Barker (69), Landay (51), Lloyd (52) and Natelson (64) and their coworkers found normal numbers and Masuda (81) and Gupta (50) and their coworkers found decreased numbers of NK cells. Despite the discrepancy in total numbers of NK cells measured by different groups, Caligiuri (82) and Morrison (80) and their coworkers found an increased proportion of CD56+CD3+ T cells, which may account for the decreased natural killer (NK) cell cytotoxic activity seen in several studies of CFS patients. Morrison and coworkers (80) also found a decreased percentage of CD56+Fcgamma receptor+ NK cells, which suggests a reduced capacity for antibody-dependent cellular toxicity.

Neutrophils

Previously described relationships in healthy women between basal circulating neutrophil numbers and plasma progesterone concentrations and between exercise-induced neutrophilia and urinary cortisol and plasma creatine kinase concentrations were not observed in CFS women, observations which suggest that normal endocrine influences on the circulating neutrophil pool may be disrupted in CFS patients (83).

IMMUNE CELL FUNCTION

T and B Lymphocytes

Depressed responses to phytohemagglutinin (PHA) and pokeweed mitogen (PWM), an indication of dysfunction in cellular immunity, were found in the CFS patients studied by most teams (45-49,52,54, 56,57,70,84,85) while Mawle and coworkers (60) found no change. Gupta and coworkers (50) found that the lymphocyte DNA synthesis in response to PHA, PWM and concanavalin A was normal in CFS patinets, but the response to soluble antigens (mumps, *E. coli*) was significantly reduced. Roberts and colleagues (42) found that PWM lymphoproliferative response is associated with Rh status among healthy controls but not among CFS patients and recommended to control future studies for Rh status. In terms of the functional implications of decreased lymphoproliferative activities in CFS, Hassan and coworkers (70) reported that PHA proliferative responses were lower in patients with poor emotional and mental health scores, and the anti-CD3/anti-CD28 response was low in those with low general health perception scores. T-cell dysfunction in CFS patients has been suggested to result from decreased surface expression of CD3, an important component of the T-cell receptor complex (86) and Barker and coworkers (69) found no significant increase in the mean proliferation of peripheral blood cells when stimulated with anti-CD3 antibody.

In terms of B-cell function, spontaneous and mitogen-induced immunoglobulin synthesis is also affected as discussed later. Despite these deficits in B-cell function, stimulation with allergens provides differential lymphocyte responsiveness. Greater *in vitro* lymphocyte responses to specific allergens, greater baseline levels of lymphocyte incorporation of tritiated thymidine, and an increased number of immunoglobulin E-bearing B and T lymphocytes have been reported (87,88). Elevation in levels of certain cytokines, such as IL-4, IL-5 and IL-6 may underlie the latter effects as discussed later.

In a sample of 65 CFS patients, we observed that decreased lymphoproliferative responses to PHA and PWM were associated with increased cognitive difficulties and greater SIP physicial illness burden (89).

Another area of research in CFS is that of apoptosis, the process of programmed cell death, which is regulated by several genes including Bax and Bcl-2. The Bcl-2 protein forms a heterodimer with Bax that inhibits apoptosis, whereas the Bax-Bax homodimer promotes it. A report by Hassan and coworkers (70) on surface and intracellular immunologic and apoptotic markers and functional lymphocyte assays after stimulation with anti-CD3/anti-CD28 antibodies or PHA in 44

CFS patients revealed increased expression of the apoptosis repressor ratio of bcl-2/bax in both CD4 and CD8. However, recent evidence indicates that induction of apoptosis might be mediated in a dysregulated immune system, such as that present in CFS, by the upregulation of growth inhibitory cytokines. In this respect, Vojdani and colleagues (90) found an increased apoptotic cell population in CFS individuals as compared to healthy controls. The increased apoptotic subpopulation in CFS individuals was accompanied by an abnormal cell arrest in the S phase and the G2/M boundary of the cell cycle as compared to the control group. In addition, CFS individuals exhibited enhanced mRNA and protein levels of the IFN-induced protein kinase RNA (PKR) product as compared to healthy controls. In 50% of the CFS samples treated with 2-aminopurine (a potent inhibitor of PKR) the apoptotic population was reduced by more then 50%. PKR-mediated apoptosis may thus contribute to the pathogenesis and the fatigue symptomatology associated with CFS. See and colleagues (91) found that addition of a glyconutrient compound (dietary supplement that supplies the crucial eight monosaccharides required for synthesis of glycoproteins) to peripheral blood cells of CFS patients *in vitro* significantly decreased the percentage of apoptotic cells (all three parameters were deficient at baseline).

In contrast to the studies described above, Swanink and coworkers (71) found no obvious difference in apoptosis in leukocyte cultures from CFS patients.

Natural Killer Cells

Several studies revealed impaired NK cell function in CFS patients as assessed by cytotoxic activity against K562 cells (45,56,58,69,82, 92-95) and a decreased number of CD56+CD3− lymphocytes (80,82). A study by Levine and coworkers (96) on NK cell activity in a family with members who had developed CFS as adults, as compared to those who had not, documented low NK cell activity in 6/8 cases and in 4/12 unaffected family members. Two of the offspring of the CFS cases had pediatric malignancies. Based on these observations, the authors suggested that the low NK cell activity in this family may be a result of a genetically determined immunologic abnormality predisposing to CFS and cancer. Gold and colleagues (97) were the only group to find elevated NK cell activity among the CFS patients they studied while Mawle and colleagues (60) found no change in NK cell function.

The changes in NK cell cytotoxic activity found by most groups could be related to several findings: 1. CD56+CD3− cells are the lymphoid subset with highest NK cell activity; and a decrease in their representation is expected to lower the value for the NK cell activity per effector cells; 2. The reduction in CD4+CD45+ T cells described previously may also result in decreased induction of suppressor/cytotoxic T cells; and 3. Reduced NK cell activity may be associated with deficiencies in the production of IL-2 and interferon (IFN)-gamma by T cells or in the ability of NK cells to respond to these lymphokines. In the terms of the latter possibility, Buchwald and Komaroff (55) found that stimulation with IL-2 failed to result in improvement of cytolytic activity in many patients with CFS.

Poor NK cell function may also be related to the finding of an impaired ability of lymphocytes from CFS patients to produce IFN-gamma in response to mitogenic stimuli (56,92). Although one study reported elevated IFN-gamma production (98) and another demonstrated normal production (99), the inability of lymphocytes from CFS patients to produce IFN-gamma found by Klimas (56), Kibler (92) and Visser (100) and their associates might represent a cellular exhaustion as a consequence of persistent viral stimulus. The latter postulate is supported by Morag (101) and Straus (45) and their colleagues' finding of elevated levels of leukocyte $2'5'$-oligoadenylate synthetase, an IFN-inducible enzyme, in lymphocytes of CFS patients. Furthermore, the lack of IFN-gamma production in CFS patients may be responsible for the impaired activation of immunoregulatory circuits, which in turn facilitates the reactivation and progression of viral infections. In this respect, Lusso and associates (102) described the prevention of intercellular spread of EBV mediated by the IFN released as a consequence of cellular response, and Borysiewicz and co-workers (49) described normal NK cell activity but reduced EBV-specific cytotoxic T-cell activity in their CFS patients. Reactivation/replication of a latent virus (such as Epstein Barr virus) secondary to decreased NK cell activity has also been proposed to modulate the immune system to induce CFS (103).

More recent research has provided alternative explanations for the decreased NK cell activity observed in CFS. A study by Ogawa and coworkers (104) revealed a possible dysfunction in the nitric oxide (NO)-mediated NK cell activation in CFS patients based on the observations that 24 hours treatment of NK cells with L-Arginine (L-Arg), one of the essential amino acids, enhanced NK cell activity in controls but not CFS patients. Although the expression of inducible NO synthase (iNOS) (the enzyme involved in the synthesis of NO from L-Arg) transcripts in peripheral blood mononuclear cells was not significantly different between healthy control subjects and CFS patients, and incubation with S-nitroso-N-acetyl-penicillamine, an NO donor, stimulated NK cell activity in healthy control subjects but not in CFS patients. See and coworkers (1991) reported that addition *in vitro* of a glyconutrient compound (dietary supplement that supplies the crucial eight monosaccharides required for synthesis of glycoproteins) to peripheral blood cells from CFS patients significantly enhanced natural killer cell activity, increased the expression of the glycoproteins CD5, CD8 and CD11a, and decreased the percentage of apoptotic cells, parameters which were all deficient at baseline. The latter observation would be consistent with a defect in glycoprotein synthesis.

See and Tilles (105) treated 30 CFS patients IFN-alpha 2a or placebo in a double-blind crossover study. Outcome was evaluated by NK cell function, lymphocyte proliferation to mitogens and soluble antigens, CD4/CD8 counts and a 10 item Quality of Life (QOL) survey. Although mean NK function rose with 12 weeks of IFN therapy, there was no significant change in the other immunologic parameters or QOL scores. When the 26 patients who completed the study were stratified according to their baseline NK cell function and lymphocyte proliferation, 4 groups were identified: 3 patients had normal NK cell function and lymphocyte proliferation when compared to normal, healthy controls, 9 had isolated deficiency in lymphocyte proliferation, 7 had diminished NK function only, and 7 had abnormalities for both parameters. QOL scores were not significantly different for the four groups at baseline. After 12 weeks of interferon therapy, QOL score significantly improved in each of the seven patients with isolated NK cell dysfunction compared to baseline. In these patients the mean NK cell function increased. Significant improvement was not recorded for QOL in the other three groups. Thus, therapy with IFN-alpha has a significant effect on the QOL of that subgroup of patients with CFS manifesting an isolated decrease in NK cell function.

Pursuing the hypothesis that the low-grade fever and fatigue in low NK syndrome (LNKS)–a condition resembling CFS in many but not all ways (57,106)–might be abrogated by interventions that normalize NK functioning, one group has tested the effects of immunopotentiators with patients diagnosed with LNKS. They found in single-blind trials (contents of medication were not revealed to patients) that while the administration of antipyretics, non-steroidal anti-inflammatory drugs or antibiotics had no detectable effects on fever, lentinan, a glucon extracted from Japanese mushrooms improved clinical symptoms and increased NKCC and antibody-dependent cellular cytotoxicity (ADCC) in patients with LNKS (107). Although preliminary, this is one of the only studies to document parallel improvement in CFS-like clinical symptoms and NKCC following an experimental manipulation. However, this study did not focus specifically on CDC-diagnosed CFS patients.

Monocytes

Prieto and coauthors (108) found significant monocyte dysfunction in patients with CFS, such as reduced display of vimentin, phagocytosis index, and surface expression of HLA-DR. These deficits responded to naloxone treatment, which suggests that increased interaction of endogenous opioids with monocyte receptors might account for the monocyte dysfunction. Gupta and coworkers (109) found that monocytes from CFS patients display an increased density of ICAM-1 and LFA-1, but showed decreased enhancing response to recombinant IFN-gamma *in vitro*. In contrast to the latter studies, Barker and coworkers (69) did not find abnormalities in superoxide anion production and phagocytosis in CFS patients. Moreover, lack of a consistent elevation of neopterin, a macrophage activation marker (see later discussion), suggests that monocytes do not appear to account for the imbalances in IL-1 described below.

Eosinophils

Conti and colleagues (110) provided evidence for eosinophil activation in CFS by demonstrating elevated serum levels of eosinophil cationic protein (ECP). In the CFS population they studied, the prevalence of RAST positivity to one or more allergens was 77%, while no control showed positive RAST. Twelve of the 14 CFS patients with increased ECP serum levels were RAST-positive. However, CFS RAST-positive patients had no significantly higher ECP serum levels than CFS RAST-negative patients. It remains to be determined whether eosinophil activation has a pathogenetic role in CFS or whether a common immunologic background may exist for both atopy and CFS.

Although a higher prevalence of allergy (111) and delayed type hypersensitivity (52,54) can be detected in CFS patients, a trial with antihistamine treatment did not provide significant improvement (112) and other authors such as Mawle and coworkers (60) found no significant difference in the incidence of delayed type hypersensitivity and allergic responses among CFS patients. Baraniuk and coworkers (113,114) found that 30% of CFS patients had positive skin tests suggesting the potential for allergic rhinitis complaints, and 46% had non-allergic rhinitis and suggested that while atopy may coexist in some CFS subjects, it is unlikely that it plays a causal role in CFS pathogenesis. Borish and coworkers (115) proposed that in at least a large subgroup of subjects with CFS with allergies, the concomitant influences of immune activation brought on by allergic inflammation in an individual with the appropriate psychologic profile may interact to produce the symptoms of CFS, and Borok (116) suggested that food intolerance, in a genetically predisposed group of people, causes symptoms akin to both the major and minor criteria of CFS and it should be screened for to avoid confusion. Although the controversy of atopy and CFS continues, it may be possible that these two conditions share some common denominators that are worth pursuing particularly in light of the proposed Th2 cytokine predominant pattern.

CYTOKINES AND OTHER SOLUBLE IMMUNE MEDIATORS

Stimulated lymphoid cells either express or induce the expression in other cells of a heterogeneous group of soluble mediators that exhibit either effector or regulatory functions. These soluble mediators include cytokines, hormones, and neurotransmitters, which in turn affect immune function and may underlie many of the pathological manifestations seen in CFS (41). The studies of cytokines in CFS have been done in the peripheral blood compartment and a recent review by Vollmer-Conna and coworkers (117) on the immunopathogenesis of CFS concludes that neuropsychiatric symptoms in CFS patients may be more closely related to disordered cytokine production by glial cells within the CNS than to circulating cytokines. The hypothesis that expression of proinflammatory cytokines within the CNS plays a role in the pathogenesis of immunologically-mediated fatigue is underscored by the study by Sheng and coworkers (118) who, using two strains of mice with differential patterns of cytokine expression in response to an injection challenge with *Corynebacterium parvum,* demonstrated that elevated IL-1 and TNF cytokine mRNA expression in the central nervous system corresponded to development of fatigue. Injection of antibodies specific to either IL-1 or TNF did not alter immunologically induced fatigue, suggesting a lack of involvement of these cytokines produced outside of the CNS. We will nonetheless describe the potential implications of the cytokine imbalances detected in peripheral blood to physiological and psychological functions.

Cytokines

The decreased NK cell cytotoxic and lymphoproliferative activities and increased allergic and autoimmune manifestations in CFS would be compatible with the hypothesis that the immune system of affected individuals is biased towards a Th2 type, or humoral immunity-oriented cytokine pattern (119). The factors that could lead to a Th2 shift and to mood changes associated with immunoendocrine changes among CFS patients are unknown. Vaccines and stressful stimuli have been shown to lead to long-term, non-specific shifts in cytokine balance. Therapeutic regimens that induce a systemic Th1 bias are being tested including repeated stimulation with bacterial antigens or poly (I)-poly (C12U) (120) and *ex vivo* activation of lymph node cells (121).

Interleukin-1 (IL-1) and Soluble IL-1 Receptors

IL-1 is the term for two distinct cytokines–IL-1α and IL-1 β–that share the same cell-surface receptors and biological activities (122,123). One study of CFS patients (124) found elevated levels of serum IL-1 alpha but not of plasma IL-1 beta in 17% of patients studied. When the cohort was examined as to severity of symptoms, it was noted that the top quartile in terms of disability had the highest level of IL-1. Curiously, use of reverse transcriptase-coupled polymerase chain reaction (RT-PCR) revealed IL-1β but not IL-1α messenger RNA (mRNA) in peripheral blood mononuclear cells (PBMCs) of several CFS patients with highly elevated levels of IL-1α. RT-PCR of fractionated cell populations showed that lymphocytes accounted for the IL-1β mRNA detected in PBMCs. No IL-1 mRNA was apparent in control subjects.

That IL-1α mRNA was not detectable by RT-PCR in either PBMCs or granulocytes suggests that serum IL-1α in CFS patients is probably derived from a source other than peripheral blood cells. Other potential sources are tissue macrophages, endothelial cells, lymph node cells, fibroblasts, central nervous system microglia, astrocytes, and dermal dendritic cells (122).

Linde and coworkers (125) found significantly higher levels of IL-1 alpha in CFS and mononucleosis patients but Lloyd (52), Peakman (72) and Rasmussen (126) and their coworkers found no difference. Five studies, in addition to one described above by Patarca and colleagues (124) found no difference in the levels of IL-1 beta in CFS patients (72,125-128).

The signs and symptoms of CFS, which include fatigue, myalgia, and low-grade fever, are similar to those experienced by patients infused with cytokines such as interleukin-1. Elevated serum levels of IL-1α found in a significant number of CFS patients could underlie several of the clinical symptoms. IL-1 can gain access to the brain through the preoptic nucleus of the hypothalamus, where it induces fever and the release of adrenocorticotropin hormone (ACTH)-releasing factor (129-132), which in turn would lead to release of ACTH and cortisol. The observation that cortisol levels tend to be low in CFS patients regardless of IL-1α levels suggests a role of a defective hypothalamic feedback loop in the pathogenesis of CFS. The presence of such a defect has been documented in Lewis rats, which are particularly susceptible to the induction of a variety of inflammatory and autoimmune diseases and exhibit reduced levels of ACTH-releasing hormone, ACTH and cortisol in response to IL-1.

Besides its effects on the HPA axis, IL-1 has other effects on the pituitary; it has been shown to augment release of prolactin and growth hormone and to inhibit release of thyrotropin and luteinizing hormone (133,134). The growth hormone deficiency state associated with CFS may also be a reflection of the defect in hypothalamic feedback loop which renders it inadequately responsive to IL-1.

IL-1 and tumor necrosis factor (TNF) provoke slow-wave sleep when placed in the lateral ventricles of experimental animals (135). The inordinate fatigue, lassitude, and excessive sleepiness associated with CFS (136,137) could well be a consequence of the direct action of these cytokines on neurons. Neurotoxic effects due to chronic over-expression of IL-1α and/or β of S100–a small (10KDa), soluble calcium-binding protein that is synthesized and released by astroglia (138)–have been proposed to underlie progressive neurological degeneration in Alzheimer's disease (139).

IL-1 induces prostaglandin (PGE_2, PGI_2) synthesis by endothelial and smooth muscle cells (140). These substances are potent vasodilators, and IL-1 administration in animals and humans produces significant hypotension. IL-1 has a natriuretic effect (141) and may affect plasma volume.

Gulick and colleagues (142) showed that IL-1 and TNF inhibit β-adrenergic agonist-mediated cardiac myocyte contractility in cultures and intracellular accumulation of cyclic adenosine monophosphate. Cytokine imbalances may, therefore, also underlie the cardiovascular manifestations of CFS.

Chronic fatigue syndrome is a condition that affects women in disproportionate numbers, and that is often exacerbated in the premenstrual period and following physical exertion. Cannon and coworkers (143) found that isolated peripheral blood mononuclear cells from healthy women, but not CFS patients, exhibited significant menstrual cycle-related differences in IL-1 beta secretion that were related to estradiol and progesterone levels. IL-1Ra secretion for CFS patients was twofold higher than controls during the follicular phase, but luteal-phase levels were similar between groups. In both phases of the menstrual cycle, IL-1sRII release was significantly higher for CFS patients compared to controls. The only changes that might be attributable to exertion occurred in the control subjects during the follicular phase, who exhibited an increase in IL-1 beta secretion 48 hr after the stress. These results suggest that an abnormality exists in IL-1 beta secretion in CFS patients that may be related to altered sensitivity to estradiol and progesterone. Furthermore, the increased release of IL-1Ra and sIL-1RII by cells from CFS patients is consistent with the hypothesis that CFS is associated with chronic, low-level activation of the immune system.

In contrast to the studies described above, Swanink and coworkers (71) found no obvious difference in the levels of circulating cytokines, and *ex vivo* production of IL-1 alpha and IL-1 receptor antagonist. Although endotoxin-stimulated *ex vivo* production of tumor necrosis factor-alpha and IL-beta was significantly lower in CFS, none of the immunologic test results correlated with fatigue severity or psychologic well-being scores. Swanink and coworkers (71) concluded that these immunologic tests cannot be used as diagnostic tools in individual CFS patients.

Tumor Necrosis Factors (TNFs) and Soluble TNF-Receptors

TNF-alpha and TNF-beta are cytokines produced on lymphoid cell activation (144). Twenty-eight percent of CFS patients studied by Patarca and colleagues (124) had elevations in serum levels of TNF-alpha and TNF-beta usually with elevation in serum levels of IL-1 or sIL-2R. TNF-alpha expression in CFS patients is also evident at the mRNA level, which suggests *de novo* synthesis rather than release of a preformed inducible surface TNF-alpha protein upon activation of monocytes and CD4+ T cells (145). The levels of spontaneously (unstimulated) produced TNF-alpha by non-adherent lymphocytes were also significantly increased as compared to simultaneously studied matched controls by Gupta and colleagues (109). TNF-alpha may be associated with CNS pathology because it has been associated with demyelination and may also lead to loss of appetite (144,146). A study by Dreisbach and coworkers (147) suggests that TNF-alpha may be involved in the pathogenesis of post-dialysis fatigue. In contrast to the studies discussed above, Lloyd et al. (52) found no difference in the levels of TNF-alpha or -beta in CFS patients and Rasmussen et al. (126) and Peakman et al. (72) found no differences in the levels of TNF-alpha and -beta, respectively. The latter discrepancies are likely due to the fact that TNF levels decrease precipitously if the serum or plasma is not frozen within 30 minutes from collection (61).

TNF-alpha's proinflammatory effects may be mediated by induction of gene expression for neutrophil activating protein-1 and macrophage inflammatory proteins resulting in neutrophil migration and degranulation (148). Thus, it is reasonable that TNF elevations may also be associated with markers of macrophage activation such as serum neopterin (see below). Among patients studied in our laboratory, we found that illness burden scores were significantly positively correlated with elevated TNF-alpha serum levels.

CFS patients have higher levels of sTNF-RI or sCD120a and sTNF-RII or sCD120b (24,25). Levels of sTNF-Rs are negatively correlated with NK cell cytotoxic and lymphoproliferative activities in CFS, an observation that is consistent with the activities of these soluble mediators.

Interleukin-2 (IL-2) and Soluble IL-2 Receptor

IL-2, formerly termed "T-cell growth factor," is a glycosylated protein produced by T lymphocytes after mitogenic or antigenic stimulation (149). IL-2 acts as a growth factor (150) and promoted proliferation of T cell (151) and, under particular conditions, of B cells and macrophages (152,153).

Although serum IL-2 levels were found to be elevated in CFS patients compared with control individuals in one study (154), decreased levels were reported in two other studies (92,97) and no difference was reported in three studies (124,125,128). Rasmussen and coworkers (126) reported a higher production of IL-2 by stimulated peripheral blood cells from CFS patients as compared to controls. Cheney and coworkers (154) found no obvious relation between IL-2 serum levels and severity or duration of illness in CFS.

Elevated levels of sIL-2R, a marker of lymphoid cell activation, have been found in a number of pathological conditions including viral infections, autoimmune diseases, and lymphoproliferative and hematological malignancies (155,156). Twelve percent of CFS patients studied by Patarca and coworkers (124) had elevated levels of sIL-2R. The latter observation is consistent with the increased proportion of activated T cells and the reduced levels of IL-2 or decreased NK cell cytotoxic activity found in several studies of CFS patients discussed above. Linde and coworkers (125) found no elevation in sIL-2R levels in CFS patients.

Interleukin-4 (IL-4)

Visser and colleagues (100) reported that although CD4 T cells from CFS patients produce less interferon-gamma than cells from controls, IL-4 production and cell proliferation are comparable. With CD4 T cells from CFS patients (compared with cells from controls), a 10- to 20-fold lower desamethasone (DEX) concentration was needed to achieve 50% inhibition of IL-4 production and proliferation, indicating an increased sensitivity to DEX in CFS patients. In contrast to IL-4, interferon-gamma production in patients and controls was equally sensitive to DEX. A differential sensitivity of cytokines or CD4 T cell subsets to glucocorticoids might explain an altered immunologic function in CFS patients.

IL-4 acts as a growth factor for various types of lymphoid cells, including B, T, and cytotoxic T cells (157), and has been shown to be involved in immunoglobulin isotype selection *in vivo* (158). Activated T cells are the major source of IL-4 production, but mast cells can also produce it, and IL-4 has been associated with allergic and autoimmune reactions (157). It is also noteworthy that many of the effects of IL-4 are antagonized by IFN-gamma, and the decreased production of the latter may underlie a predominance of IL-4 over IFN-gamma effects.

Interleukin-6 (IL-6) and Soluble IL-6 Receptor

The levels of spontaneously produced IL-6 by both adherent monocytes and non-adherent lymphocytes were significantly increased in CFS patients as compared to controls (109). The abnormality of IL-6 was also observed at mRNA level. In terms of circulating IL-6, Buchwald and coworkers (23) found that IL-6 was elevated among febrile CFS patients compared to those without this finding and therefore considered it an epiphenomenon possibly secondary to infection. Chao and coworkers (159,160) also found elevated levels of IL-6 in CFS patients, but five other groups found no difference (23,52,72,94,125).

Most of the cell types that produce IL-6 so in response to stimuli such as IL-1 and TNF, among others (161). Excessive IL-6 production has been associated with polyclonal B-cell activation, resulting in hypergammaglogulinemia and auto antibody production (162). As is the case with IL-4, IL-6 may contribute to activation of CD5-bearing B cells, leading to autoimmune manifestations. IL-6 also synergizes with IL-1 in inflammatory reactions and may exacerbate many of the features described previously for IL-1.

Study of cytokine production by stimulated peripheral blood mononuclear cells from patients with a closely related syndrome to CFS, the post-Q-fever fatigue syndrome (QFS) (inappropriate fatigue, myalgia and arthralgia, night sweats, changes in mood and sleep patterns following about 20% of laboratory-proven, acute primary Q-fever cases), showed an accentuated release of IL-6 which was significantly in excess of medians for all four control groups (resolving QFS, acute primary Q-fever without subsequent QFS, healthy Q-fever vaccinees and healthy controls). Levels of induced IL-6 significantly correlated with total symptom scores and scores for other key symptoms (163).

CFS patients have higher levels of sIL-6R (24) and sIL-6R enhances the effects of IL-6.

Interleukin-10 (IL-10)

A study by Gupta and coworkers (109) revealed that spontaneously produced IL-10 by both adherent monocytes and non-adherent lymphocytes and by PHA-activated non-adherent monocytes were decreased. IL-10 is part of the Th2-type response.

Interferons (IFNs)

The IFNs comprise a multigenic family with pleiotropic properties and diverse cellular origin. Data from six studies indicate that circulating IFNs are present in 3% or less of patients studied (45,48,49,55,57, 164,165).

Peripheral blood cells from children affected by postviral fatigue syndrome produced more IFN-alpha than those from controls. In line with latter observation, Vojdani and colleagues (90) found elevated IFN-alpha levels in CFS patients but Linde (125) and Straus (128) and their coworkers found no difference. Fatigue occurs in more than 70% of patients treated with IFN-alpha and it may be associated with the development of immune-mediated endocrine diseases, in particular hypothryoidism and hypothalamic-pituitary-adrenal axis-related hormonal deficiencies, in these patients (166,167). IFN-alpha therapy-associated fatigue is often the dominant dose-limiting side effect, worsening with continued therapy, and accompanied by significant depression. Decreases in mental information processing speeds, verbal memory, and executive functions have also been reported at therapeutic doses of IFN-alpha (168). Although the direct cause of IFN-alpha-induced fatigue is unknown, it is possible that neuromuscular fatigue, similar to that observed in patients with postpolio syndrome, may also be one component of this syndrome. The induction of proinflammatory cytokines observed in patients treated with IFN-alpha is consistent with a possible mechanism of neuromuscular pathology that could manifest as fatigue. A study by Davis and colleagues (169) also revealed that IFN-alpha/beta is at least partially responsible for the early fatigue induced by polyI:C during prolonged treadmill running in mice.

IFN-gamma is an immunoregulatory substance, enhancing both cellular antigen presentation to lymphocytes (170) and NK cell cytotoxicity (171) and causing inhibition of suppressor T lymphocyte activity (172). Two groups have found impaired IFN-gamma production on mitogenic stimulation of peripheral blood mononuclear cells from CFS patients (56,100) and one group (52) found increased production. In contrast with the findings on lymphocyte activation, four groups reported no difference in the levels of circulating IFN-gamma (72,100, 125,128). These results are in favor of the Th2 shift described previously, a shift that is not apparent at the level of circulating cytokines.

Tumor Growth Factor-Beta (TGF-Beta)

A study by Bennett and coworkers (173) found that patients with CFS had significantly higher levels of bioactive TGF-beta levels compared to healthy controls and to patients with various diseases known to be associated with immunologic abnormalities and/or pathologic fatigue: major depression, systemic lupus erythematosis (SLE), and multiple sclerosis (MS) of both the relapsing/remitting (R/R) and the chronic progressive (CP) types. A total of three studies supports the finding of elevated levels of TGF-beta among CFS patients.

Beta-2 Microglobulin

Three studies found elevated levels of beta-2 microglobulin in patients with CFS (23-25) and one study found no difference (159). Beta-2 microglobulin is a marker of immune activation.

Neopterin

Neopterin is a metabolite produced during the utilization of guanosine triphosphate, and increased production of neopterin is associated with macrophage activation by IFN gamma (174,175). Neopterin is a presumed primate homolog of nitric oxide, which activated guanylate cyclase and is involved in neurotransmission, vasodilation, neurotoxicity, inhibition of platelet aggregation, the antiproliferative action of cytokines, and reduction of oxidative stress (176,177). Neopterin derivatives belong to the cytotoxic arsenal of the activated human macrophage and, in high doses, enhance oxidative stress through enhancemente of radical-mediated effector functions and programmed cell death by TNF-alpha, while having an opposite effect at low doses (176,178). Buchwald (23) and Chao (159,160) and their coworkers found elevated levels of neopterin in CFS patients, while Linde (125) and Patarca (124) and their coworkers found no difference. A report of nine CFS cases showed significantly elevated serum neopterin levels in association with high Cognitive Difficulty Scale (CDS) scores (89,179) and neopterin levels have been shown to correlate with levels of many other mediators that have been found to be dysregulated in CFS including members of the TNF family (23,41,124). In terms of neurotoxicity, serum neopterin and tryptophan concentrations correlate among cancer and AIDS patients, an observation which can be accounted for by activity of indoleamine 2,3-dioxygenase, a tryptophan-degrading enzyme (180,181). The latter enzyme also converts L-tryptophan to L-kynurenine, kynurenic acid and quinolinic acid (QUIN). QUIN is a neurotoxic metabolite that accumulates within the central nervous system following immune activation and is also a sensitive marker for the presence of immune activation within the CNS (182-184). Direct conversion of L-tryptophan into QUIN by brain tissue occurs in conditions of CNS inflammation, but not by normal brain tissue. Macrophage infiltrates, and perhaps microglia, are important sources of QUIN, an observation which is consistent with the results of inoculation of poliovirus directly into the spinal cord of rhesus macaques, resulting in increased CSF levels of both QUIN and neopterin (182,185). Elevated serum levels of neopterin correlate with the presence of brain lesions and with neurologic and psychiatric symptoms in patients with AIDS dementia complex (179, 186). It is worth noting in this context that Buchwald and colleagues (187) found subcortical lesions consistent with edema and demyelination by magnetic resonance scans in 78% of CFS patients as compared to 20% of controls.

Soluble CD8 (sCD8)

Linde and coworkers (125) found no elevation of sCD8 in CFS patients.

Soluble ICAM-1 (sICAM-1)

Patarca and coworkers (24) found higher levels of sICAM-1 in CFS patients, an observation which is consistent with the higher expresion of ICAM-1 in monocytes of CFS patients reported by Gupta and coworkers (50).

Immunoglobulins

Spontaneous and mitogen-induced immunoglobulin synthesis is depressed in 10% of patients with CFS (49,188,189). The latter decrease may be a result of an increased T-cell suppression of immunoglobulin synthesis, because a similar effect is obtained *in vitro* when using normal allogeneic B cells (189). This inhibitory effect may also account for the reported difficulty in establishing spontaneous outgrowth of EBV-transformed B-cell lines from cells from CFS patients (45,55,189). The depletion of the CD4+CD45RA+ lymphocyte subset in the studies by Klimas et al. (56) and Franco and colleagues (65) may be associated with alteration in B-cell regulation.

In twelve studies, CFS patients were found to have decreased amounts of immunoglobulins of the G, A, M, or D classes (45,48,54, 55,58,126,189-194); in five studies no difference was found (50,52, 60,64,72); and in one study IgG levels were elevated while IgA levels were normal (207). IgG subclass deficiency, particularly of the opsonins IgG1 or IgG3, can be demonstrated in a substantial percentage of CFS patients (54,56,59,191,194,195), and for a subset of these, immunoglobulin replacement therapy may be beneficial (196-199) albeit controversial (199). Bennett and coworkers (200) also failed to find immunoglobulin subclass deficiencies in CFS patients.

Autoantibodies

Konstantinov and colleagues (202) found that approximately 52% of sera from CFS patients react with nuclear envelope antigens. Some sera immunoprecipitated nuclear envelope protein lamin B1, an observation which underscores an autoimmune component in CFS (203). von Mikecz and colleagues (204) found a high frequency (83%) of autoantibodies to insoluble cellular antigens (vimentin and lamin B1) in CFS, a unique feature which might help to distinguish CFS from other rheumatic autoimmune diseases. Another finding that underscores a possible autoimmune etiology is the significant association between CFS and the presence of HLA-DQ3 reported by Keller and colleagues (205).

The presence of rheumatoid factor (45-48,85,108,192,206), antinuclear antibodies (45-48,85,97,108,193,204,207,208), antithyroid antibodies (84,85,209), anti-smooth-muscle antibodies (84), antigliadin, cold agglutinins, cryoglobulins, and false serological positivity for syphilis (45,84) have also been reported. No circulating antimuscle and anti-CNS antibodies were found in 10 CFS patients (210) and Rasmussen and coworkers (126) found no significant differences in the number of positive tests for autoantibodies in CFS patients.

Circulating Immune Complexes

Elevated levels of immune complexes have been reported in four studies (45,49,84,207) while the studies by Natelson (64) and Mawle (60) and their coworkers revealed no abnormality in the level of circulating immune complexes (i.e., Raji cell and C1q binding). Depressed levels of complement have also been reported in 0% to 25% of patients (45,49,60,64,84). Buchwald and coworkers (23) found elevated levels of C-reactive protein among CFS patients.

EXPERIMENTAL THERAPY RESULTS IN AN APPARENT SHIFT IN THE TYPE 1 TO TYPE 2 CYTOKINE PATTERN IN CFS PATIENTS

Our group completed a safety and feasibility study using lymph node extraction, *ex vivo* cell culture, followed by autologous cell reinfusion as a treatment strategy in CFS patients (121). Lymph nodes were obtained from patients who met the current case definition for CFS and the following inclusion criteria: a history of acute onset; a Karnofsky score < 80; evidence of immune dysfunction in 3 or more of the following: > 1 S.D. above controls for elevated sTNF-RI in serum, elevated sTNF-RI in PHA-stimulated blood culture or elevated IL-5 in PHA-stimulated blood culture; or lymphocyte activation (CD2+CD26+ cells > 50%); or low NK cytotoxic activity (< 20%). The lymph node cells were cultured for 10 to 12 days with anti-CD3 and IL-12. These cells were then reinfused into the donor who was monitored for safety and possible clinical benefit. There were no adverse events noted in this Phase 1 clinical trial. Of 13 subjects, two had palpable lymph nodes that proved fibrotic with no viable cells. Of the remaining 11 subjects, all successfully underwent expansion and re-infusion. In some of the patients, there was an elevation in the expression of IL-2 receptor on CD4 T cells in the weeks following the reinfusion. There was a significant decrease in IL-5 production by PHA-stimulated blood cultures observed at 1 week which persisted for several weeks post-infusion. Levels of PHA-induced IFN-gamma did not change. There was a trend towards a decrease in the ration of IFN-gamma/IL-5 starting at week 1 and persisting at least 12 weeks. Of the 11 subjects, 9 had significant cognitive improvement, other measures of severity of illness also trended towards improvement. The lack of adverse effects from this experimental approach to immuno-modulation in CFS and the favorable clinical and immunologic results observed in the small number of patients studied suggest that further clinical trials are warranted.

STRESSORS, CYTOKINES, AND SYMPTOMS

One of our models of CFS holds that the interaction of psychologi-cal factors (distress associated with either CFS-related symptoms or other stressful life events) and immunologic dysfunction (indicated in signs of chronic overactivation with cytokine abnormalities) contrib-ute to: (a) CFS-related physical symptoms (e.g., fatigue, joint pain, cognitive difficulties, fever) and increases in illness burden; and (b) dys-function in the immune system's ability to survey viruses including latent herpesviruses (indicated in impaired NKCC). As discussed above, there is a decrease in the ratio of type 1/type 2 cytokines produced by lymphocytes *in vitro* following mitogen stimulation in CFS patients. This type of dysfunction should be expected to result in impaired immune surveillance associated with cytotoxic lymphocytes. For example, Cohen et al. (211) found an association between psycho-social stressors, immunomodulation, and the incidence and progres-sion of rhinovirus infections in healthy normals. Here, the rates of respiratory infections and clinical colds increased in a dose-response fashion with increases in psychological stress across all five of the cold viruses studied. If viruses related to upper respiratory tract infec-tions (URIs) are not well controlled by immune surveillance mecha-nisms (e.g., NKCC) in CFS patients who are exposed to stressors, then patients may suffer more frequent and protracted URIs which are accompanied by prolonged elevations in proinflammatory cytokines. Stress-associated reactivation of latent herpesviruses may also play a role in modulating the production of cytokines that underlie CFS symptom exacerbations (103,212). Alternatively, distress increases may more directly influence cytokine dysregulation by way of neu-roendocrine changes which in turn intensify physical symptoms. Importantly, for all of the possible paths, further increases in distress as a "reaction" to mounting symptoms creates a vicious cycle. Such a recursive system may act as a positive feedback loop thereby accounting for the chronic nature of CFS and its refraction to interventions that focus solely on symptom reduction.

Our conceptual model for CFS was supported by data from our laboratory showing that distress levels in response to the stressor Hurricane Andrew were positively correlated with: alterations in NK cells and elevated (compared to pre-storm values) circulating levels of the cytokines; exacerbation in CFS symptoms; and increases in Sickness Impact profile (SIP)-based illness burden scores among our CFS patients (178). We found that CFS patients living in a Hurricane exposure area (Dade County) had significantly greater severity of CFS symptom relapses (using clinician-rated fatigue levels and ability to engage in work-related activities) and significantly greater increases in illness burden as compared to age- and gender-matched CFS patients from the same clinical practice living in an adjacent geographical region that was not in the storm's path, Broward/Palm beach county. We also found that pre-post hurricane NKCC changes were associated with pre-post storm symptom severity changes including cognitive symptoms, muscle weakness, and muscle pain. These data suggested that stressor-induced decrements in NKCC were associated with greater increases in the severity of cognitive difficulties, muscle weakness and pain symptoms. A final regression analysis on NKCC indicated that appraisals in greater storm impact and low social support predicted the greatest pre-post storm decrements in NKCC. Greater optimism and social support provisions were also associated with less elevations in TNF-alpha among storm victims.

CONCLUSIONS

The data summarized herein indicate that CFS is associated with immune abnormalities that can potentially account for physio- and psychopathological symptomatology. Assessment of immune status reveals a heterogeneity among CFS patients that allows their categorization, thus systematizing the study of the interactions among immune, psychological, and physiological parameters in this disorder. The study of immune status at different levels also provides an integrated view of this complex syndrome and is opening doors for deciphering its cause and for developing rational treatment protocols. Future research should further elucidate the cellular basis for immune dysfunction in CFS and its implications. Other compartments such as the central nervous system have to be assessed using similar techniques to those used with peripheral blood. Nonetheless, the studies in peripheral blood have been providing insight into the physio- and psychopathologies of CFS.

REFERENCES

1. Shanks N, Francis D, Zalcman S, Meaney MJ, Anisman H: Alterations in central cathecolamines associated with immune responses in adult and aged mice. Brain Res 666(1):77-87, 1994.

2. Besedovsky H, del Rey A, Sorkien E, Da Prada M, Burri R, Honegger C: The immune response evokes changes in brain noradrenergic neurons. Science 221(4610):564-566, 1983.

3. Vasina IG, Frolov EP, Serebriakov NG: Sympathico-adrenal system activity in a primary immune response. Zhurnal Mikrobiologii, Epidemiologii i Imunobiologii 10(9):88-92, 1975.

4. Boranic M: The central nervous system and immunity. Lijecnicki Vjesnik 112(9-10):329-334, 1990.

5. Boranic M, Pericic D, Radacic M, Poljak-Blasi M, Sverko V, Miljenovic G: Immunological and neuroendocrine responses of rats to prolonged or repeated stress. Biomedicine & Pharmacotherapy 36(1):23-28, 1982.

6. Basso AM, Depiante-Depaoli M, Molina VA: Chronic variable stress facilitates tumoral growth: reversal by imipramine administration. Life Sciences 50(23):1789-1796, 1992.

7. Foley FW, Traugott U, LaRocca NG, Smith CR, Perlman KR, Caruso LS, Scheinberg LC: A prospective study of depression and immune dysregulation in multiple sclerosis. Arch Neurol 49(3):238-244, 1992.

8. De Souza EB: Corticotropin-releasing factor and interleukin-1 receptors in the brain-endocrine-immune axis. Role in stress response and infection. Annals of the New York Academy of Sciences 697:9-27, 1993.

9. Irwin M: Stress-induced immune suppression. Role of the autonomic nervous system. Annals of the New York Academy of Sciences 697:203-218, 1993.

10. Weiss JM, Quan N, Sundar SK: Widespread activation and consequences of interleukin-1 in the brain. Annals of the New York Academy of Sciences 741:338-357, 1994.

11. Hebert TB, Cohen S: Depression and immunity: a meta-analytic review. Psychol Bull 113:472-486, 1993.

12. Irwin M, Patterson T, Smith TL, Caldwell C, Brown SA, Gillin JC, Grant I: Reduction of immune function in life stress and depression. Biological Psychiatry 27:222-230, 1990.

13. Irwin M, Caldwell C, Smith TL, Brown S, Schuckit MA, Gillin C: Major depressive disorder, alcoholism, and reduced natural killer cell cytotoxicity. Archives of General Psychiatry 47:713-719, 1990.

14. Schleifer SJ, Keller SE, Bond RN, Cohen J, Stein M: Major depressive disorder: role of age, sex, severity and hospitalization. Achives of general Psychiatry 46:81-87, 1989.

15. Lechin F, van der Dijs B, Acosta E, Gomez F, Lechin E, Arocha L: Distal colon motility and clinical parameters in depression. J Afect Dis 5:19-26, 1983.

16. Lechin F, van der Dijs B, Gomez F, Arocha L, Acosta E, Lechin E: Distal colon motility as a predictor of antidepressant response to fenfluramine, imipramine and clomipramine. J Affect Dis 5:27-35, 1983.

17. Lechin F, van der Dijs, Jakubowicz D, et al: Effects of clonidine on blood pressure, noradrenaline, cortisol, growth hormone and prolactin plasma levels in low and high intestinal tone depressed patients. Neuroendocrinology 41:156-162, 1985.

18. Lechin F, van der Dijs B, Jakubowicz D, et al: Role of stress in the exacerbation of chronic illness: Effects of clonidine administration on blood pressure and plasma norepinephrine, cortisol, growth hormone and prolactin concentrations. Psychoneuroendocrinology 12:117-129, 1987.

19. Lechin F, van der Dijs B, Amat J, Lechin M: Central neuronal pathways involved in depressive syndrome: Experimental findings. *In* Neurochemistry and Clinical Disorders: Circuitry of Some Psychiatric and Psychosomatic Syndromes. Lechin F, van der Dijs B (eds.). Boca Raton, FL, CC press, 1989, pp. 65-89.

20. Lechin F, van der Dijs B, Lechin A, et al: Plasma neurotransmitters and cortisol in chronic illness: Role of stress. J Med 25:181-192, 1994.

21. Patarca R, Fletcher MA, Klimas NG: Immunological correlates of the chronic fatigue syndrome. *In* Chronic Fatigue Syndrome, P Goodnick, NG Klimas (eds.). Washington, American Psychiatric Press, 1992, pp. 1-21.

22. Sobel RA, Hafler DA, Castro EE, et al: The 2H4 (CD45R) antigen is selectively decreased in multiple sclerosis lesions. J Immunol 140:2210-2214, 1988.

23. Buchwald D, Wener MH, Pearlman T, Kith P: Markers of inflammation and immune activation in chronic fatigue and chronic fatigue syndrome. Journal of Rheumatology 24(2):372-6, 1997.

24. Patarca R, Klimas NG, Garcia MN, Pons H, Fletcher MA: Dysregulated expression of soluble immune mediator receptors in a subset of patients with chronic fatigue syndrome: Categorization of patients by immune status. Journal of Chronic Fatigue Syndrome 1:79-94, 1995.

25. Patarca R, Klimas NG, Sandler D, Garcia MN, Fletcher MA: Interindividual immune status variation patterns in patients with chronic fatigue syndrome: association with the tumor necrosis factor system and gender. Journal of Chronic Fatigue Syndrome 2(1):13-19, 1995.

26. Goldie AS, Fearon KCH, Ross JA, Barclay R, Jackson RE, Grant IS, Ramsay G, Blyth AS, Howie JC, The Sepsis Intervention Group. Natural cytokine antagonists and endogenous antiendotoxin core antibodies in sepsis syndrome. JAMA 274:172-177, 1995.

27. Cantor H, Boyse EA: Regulation of cellular and humoral immune responses by T-cell subclasses. Cold Spring Harbor Symp Quant Biol 41:23-32, 1977.

28. Reinherz EL, Schlossman SF: The characterization and function of human immunoregulatory T lymphocyte subsets. Immunology Today 2:6975-6979, 1981.

29. Romain P, Schlossman S: Human T lymphocyte subsets. Functional heterogeneity and surface recognition structures. J Clin Invest 74:1559-1565, 1984.

30. Calabrese JR, Kling MA, Gold PA: Alterations in immunocompetence during stress, bereavement, and depression: focus on neuroendocrine regulation. Am J Psychiatry 144:1123-1134, 1987.

31. Fletcher MA, Azen S, Adelberg B, et al: Immunophenotyping in a multicenter study: the transfusion safety experience. Clin Immunol Immunopatol 52:38-47, 1989.

32. Griffin DE: Immunologic abnormalities accompanying acute and chronic viral infections. Rev Infect Dis 13(1):S129-S133, 1991.

33. Klimas N, Patarca R, Perez G, et al: Distinctive immune abnormalities in a patient with procainamide-induced lupus and serositis. Am J Med Sci 303(2):1-6, 1992.

34. McAllister CG, Rapaport MH, Pickar D, et al: Increased numbers of CD5+ B lymphocytes in schizophrenic patients. Arch Gen Psychiatry 46:890-894, 1989.

35. Raziuddin S, Elawad ME: Immunoregulatory CD4+CD45R+ suppressor/inducer T lymphocyte subsets and impaired cell-mediated immunity in patients with Down's syndrome. Clin Exp Immunol 79:67-71, 1990.

36. Villemain F, Chatenoud L, Galinowski A, et al: Aberrant T cell-mediated immunity in untreated schizophrenic patients: deficient interleukin-2 production. Am J Psychiatry 146:609-616, 1989.

37. Herberman RB: Sources of confounding in immunologic data. Rev Infect Dis 13(1):S84-S86, 1991.

38. Lahita RG: Sex hormones and immunity. *In* Basic and Clinical Immunology, DP, Stobo JD, Fudenberg HH, et al. (eds.), Los Altos, CA, Lange, 1982, pp. 293-294.

39. Malone JL, Simms TE, Gray GC, et al: Sources of variability in repeated T-helper lymphocyte counts from human immunodeficiency virus type 1-infected patients: total lymphocyte count fluctutations and diurnal cycle are important. Journal of Acquired Immune Deficiency Syndromes 3:144-151, 1990.

40. Martin E, Muler JV, Dionel C: Disappearance of CD4 lymphocyte circadian cycles in HIV-infected patients: early event during asymptomatic infection. AIDS 2:133-134, 1988.

41. Patarca R, Sandler D, Walling J, Klimas NG, Fletcher MA: Assessment of immune mediator expression levels in biological fluids and cells: a critical appraisal. Critical Reviews in Oncogenesis 6(2):117-149, 1995.

42. Roberts TK, McGregor NR, Dunstan RH, Donohoe M, Murdoch RN, Hope D, Zhang S, Butt HL, Watkins JA, Taylor WG: Immunological and haematological parameters in patients with chronic fatigue syndrome. Journal of Chronic Fatigue Syndrome 4(4):51-66, 1998.

43. Schulte PA: Validation of biologic markers for use in research on chronic fatigue syndrome. Rev Infect Dis 13:S87-S89, 1991.

44. Whiteside TL: Cytokine measurements and interpretation in human disease. J Clin Immunol 14:327-339, 1994.

45. Straus SE, Tosato G, Armstrong G, et al: Persisting illness and fatigue in adults with evidence of Epstein-Barr virus infection. Ann Intern Med 102:7-16, 1985.

46. Jones J: Serologic and immunologic responses in chronic fatigue syndrome with emphasis on the Epstein-Barr virus. Rev Infect Dis 13(1):S26-S31, 1991.

47. Jones JF, Straus SE: Chronic Epstein-Barr virus infection. Annu Rev Med 38:195-209, 1987.

48. Jones JF, Ray G, Minnich LL, et al: Evidence for active Epstein-Barr virus infection in patients with persistent, unexplained illnesses: elevated anti-early antigen antibodies. Ann Intern Med 102:1-7, 1985.

49. Borysiewicz LK, Haworth SJ, Cohen J, et al: Epstein-Barr virus–specific immune defects in patients with persistent symptoms following infectious mononucleosis. Q J Med 58:111-121, 1986.

50. Gupta S, Vayuvegula B: A comprehensive immunological analysis in chronic fatigue syndrome. Scand J Immunol 33(3):319-327, 1991.

51. Landay AL, Jessop C, Lennette ET, Levy JA: Chronic fatigue syndrome: clinical condition associated with immune activation. Lancet 338:707-712, 1991.

52. Lloyd A, Hickie I, Hickie C, Dwyer J, Wakefield D: Cell-mediated immunity in patients with chronic fatigue syndrome, healthy controls and patients with major depression. Clin exp Immunol 87(1):76-79, 1992.

53. Tirelli U, Marotta G, Improta S, Pinto A: Immunological abnormalities in patients with chronic fatigue syndrome. Scand J Immunol 40(6):601-608, 1994.

54. Lloyd AR, Wakefield D, Boughton CR, et al: Immunological abnormalities in the chronic fatigue syndrome. Med J Aust 151:122-124, 1989.

55. Buchwald D, Komaroff AL: Review of laboratory findings for patients with chronic fatigue syndrome. Rev Infect Dis 13(1):S12-S18, 1991.

56. Klimas N, Salvato F, Morgan R, Fletcher MA: Immunologic abnormalities in chronic fatigue syndrome. J Clin Microbiol 28(6):1403-1410, 1990.

57. Aoki T, Usuda Y, Miyakashi H, et al: Low natural syndrome: clinical and immunologic features. Nat Immun Cell Growth Regul 6:116-128, 1987.

58. DuBois RE: Gamma globulin therapy for chronic mononucleosis syndrome. AIDS Res Hum Retroviruses 2(1):S191-S195, 1986.

59. Linde A, Hammarstrom L, Smith CIE: IgG subclass deficiency and chronic fatigue syndrome. Lancet 1:885-886, 1988.

60. Mawle AC, Nisenbaum R, Dobbins JG, Gary HE Jr, Stewart JA, Reyes M, Steele L, Schmid DS, Reeves WC: Immune responses associated with chronic fatigue syndrome: A case-control study. Journal of Infectious Diseases 175(1):136-141, 1997.

61. Patarca R, Goodkin K, Fletcher MA: Cryopreservation of peripheral blood mononuclear cells. *In* Manual of Clinical Laboratory Immunology, Rose NR, de Macario EC, Folds JD, Lane HC, Nakamura RM (Eds.), 1995.

62. Sandman CA, Barron JL, Nackoul KA, Fidler PL, Goldstein J: Is there a chronic fatigue syndrome (CFS) dementia. *In* The Clinical and Scientific Basis of Myalgic Encephalomyelitis/Chronic Fatigue Syndrome, Hyde B, Levine P, Goldstein J (eds.). Nightingale Research Foundation. Ottawa Canada, 1992, pp. 467-479.

63. Morimoto C, Letvin NL, Distaso JA, et al: The isolation and characterization of the human suppressor inducer T cell subset. J Immunol 134: 1508-1512, 1985.

64. Natelson BH, LaManca JJ, Denny TN, Vladutiu A, Oleske J, Hill N, Bergen MT, Korn L, Hay J: Immunologic parameters in chronic fatigue syndrome, major de-

pression, and multiple sclerosis. American Journal of Medicine 105(3A):43S-49S, 1998.

65. Franco K, Kawa HA, Doi S, et al: Remarkable depression of CD4+2H4+ T cells in severe chronic active Epstein-Barr virus infection. Scand J Immunol 26:769-773, 1987.

66. Alpert S, Kloide J, Takada S, et al: T cell regulatory disturbances in the rheumatic diseases. Rheum Dis Clin North Am 13(3):431-435, 1987.

67. Emery P, Gently KC, Mackay IR, et al: Deficiency of the suppressor inducer subset of T lymphocytes in rheumatoid arthritis. Arthitis Rheum 30: 849-856, 1987.

68. Sato K, Miyasaka N, Yamaoka K, et al: Quantitative defect of CD4+2H4+ cells in systemic lupus erythematosus and Sjogren's syndrome. Arthritis Rheum 30:1407-1411, 1987.

69. Barker E, Fujimura SF, Fadem MB, Landay AL, Levy JA: Immunologic abnormalities associated with chronic fatigue syndrome. Clin Infect Dis 18(supp 1): S136-S141, 1994.

70. Hassan IS, Bannister BA, Akbar A, Weir W, Bofill M: A study of the immunology of the chronic fatigue syndrome: Correlation of immunologic markers to health dysfunction. Clinical Immunology & Immunopathology 87(1):60-67, 1998.

71. Swanink CM, Vercoulen JH, Galama JM, Roos MT, Meyaard L, van der Ven-Jongekrijg J, de Nijs R, Bleijenberg G, Fennis JF, Miedema F, van der Meer JW: Lymphocyte subsets, apoptosis, and cytokines in patients with chronic fatigue syndrome. Journal of Infectious Diseases 173(2):460-463, 1996.

72. Peakman M, Deale A, Field R, Mahalingam M, Wessely S: Clinical improvement in chronic fatigue syndrome is not associated with lymphocyte subsets of function or activation. Clinical Immunology & Immunopathology 82(1):83-91, 1997.

73. Alviggi L, Johnson C, Hopkins PJ, et al: Pathogenesis of insulin-dependent diabetes: a role for activated T lymphocytes. Lancet 2:4-6, 1984.

74. Canonina GW, Bagnasco M, Corte G, et al: Circulating T lymphocytes in Hashimoto's disease: imbalance of subsets and presence of activated cells. Clin Immunol Immunopathol 23:616-625, 1982.

75. Jackson RA, Haynes BF, Burch WM, et al: Ia+ T cells in new onset Grave's disease. J Clin Endocrinol Metab 59:187-190, 1984.

76. Koide J: Functional property of Ia-positive T cells in peripheral blood from patients with systemic lupus erythematosus. Scand J Immunol 22:577-584, 1985.

77. Rabinowe SL, Jackson RA, Dluhy RG, et al: Ia-positive T lymphocytes in recently diagnosed idiopathic Addison's disease. Am J Med 77:597-601, 1984.

78. Helder L, Wagner S, Keller R, Klimas N, Antoni M: Markers of immune activation are associated with psychological distress in patients with CFS. Abstract, IV AACFS meeting, Cambridge, MA, 1998.

79. Casali P, Notkins AL: CD5+ B lymphocytes, polyreactive antibodies and the human B cell repertoire. Immunology Today 10:364-368, 1989.

80. Morrison LJ, Behan WH, Behan PO: Changes in natural killer cell phenotype in patients with post-viral fatigue syndrome. Clin Exp Immunol 83:441-446, 1991.

81. Masuda A, Nozoe SI, Matsuyama T, Tanaka H: Psychobehavioral and immunological characteristics of adult people with chronic fatigue and patients with chronic fatigue syndrome. Psychosom Med 56(6):516-518, 1994.

82. Caligiuri M, Murray C, Buchwald D, Levine H, Cheney P, Peterson D, Komaroff AL, Kitz J: Phenotypic and functional deficiency of natural killer cells in patients with chronic fatigue syndrome. J Immunol 139(10):3306-3313, 1987.

83. Cannon JG, Angel JB, Abad LW, O'Grady J, Lundgren N, Fagioli L, Komaroff AL: Hormonal influences on stress-induced neutrophil mobilization in health and chronic fatigue syndrome. Journal of Clinical Immunology 18(4):291-298, 1998.

84. Behan PO, Behan WHM, Bell EJ: The postviral fatigue syndrome–An analysis of the findings in 50 cases. J Infect 1985;10:211-22, 1985.

85. Tobi M, Morag A, Ravid Z, et al: Prolonged atypical illness associated with serological evidence of persistent Epstein-Barr infection. Lancet 1:61-64, 1982.

86. Subira ML, Castilla A, Civeira MP, et al: Deficient display of CD3 on lymphocytes of patients with chronic fatigue syndrome. J Infect Dis 160:165-166, 1989.

87. Olson GB, Kanaan MN, Gersuk GM, et al: Correlation between allergy and persistent Epstein-Barr virus infections in chronic active Epstein-Barr virus infected patients. J Allergy Clin Immunol 78:308-314, 1986.

88. Olson GB, Kanaan MN, Kelley LM, et al: Specific allergen-induced Epstein-barr nucler antigen-positive B cells from patients with chronic active Epstein-Barr virus infections. J Allergy Clin Immunol 78:315-320, 1986.

89. Lutgendorf S, Klimas NG, Antoni M, Brickman A, Fletcher MA: Relationships of cognitive difficulties to immune measures, depression and illness burden in chronic fatigue syndrome. Journal of Chronic Fatigue Syndrome 1(2):23-41, 1995.

90. Vojdani A, Ghoneum M, Choppa PC, Magtoto L, Lapp CW: Elevated apoptotic cell population in patients with chronic fatigue syndrome: The pivotal role of protein kinase RNA. Journal of Internal Medicine 242(6):465-478, 1997.

91. See DM, Cimoch P, Chou S, Chang J, Tilles J: The *in vitro* immunodulatory effects of glyconutrients on peripheral blood mononuclear cells of patients with chronic fatigue syndrome. Integrative Physiological & Behavioral Science 33(3): 280-287, 1998.

92. Kibler R, Lucas DO, Hicks M, et al: Immune function in hronic active Epstein-Barr virus infection. J Clin Immunol 5:46-54, 1985.

93. Ojo-Amaise EA, Conley EJ, Peters JB: Decreased natural killer cell activity is associated with severity of chronic fatigue immune deficiency syndrome. Clin Inf Dis 18:S157-S159, 1994.

94. See DM, Broumand N, Sahl L, Tilles JG: In vitro effect of echinacea and ginseng on natural killer and antibody-dependent cell cytotoxicity in healthy subjects and chronic fatigue syndrome or acquired immunodeficiency syndrome. Immunopharmacology 35:229-235, 1997.

95. Whiteside TL, Friberg D: Natural killer cells and natural killer cell activity in chronic fatigue syndrome. American Journal of Medicine 1998; 105(3A):27S-34S, 1998.

96. Levine PH, Whiteside TL, Friberg D, Bryant J, Colclough G, Herberman RB: Dysfunction of natural killer activity in a family with chronic fatigue syndrome. Clinical Immunology & Immunopathology 88(1):96-104 1998.

97. Gold D, Bowden R, Sixbey J, et al: Chronic fatigue. A prospective clinical and virologic study. JAMA 264:48-53, 1990.

98. Altman C, Larratt K, Golubjatnikov R, et al: Immunologic markers in the chronic fatigue syndrome. Clin Res 36:845A, 1988.

99. Morte S, Castilla A, Civeira M-P, Serrano M, Prieto J: Gamma-interferon and chronic fatigue syndrome. Lancet 2:623-624, 1988.

100. Visser J, Blauw B, Hinloopen B, Brommer E, de Kloet ER, Kluft C, Nagel-kerken L: CD4 T lymphocytes from patients with chronic fatigue syndrome have decreased interferon-gamma production and increased sensitivity to dexamethasone. Journal of Infectious Diseases 177(2):451-454, 1998.

101. Morag A, Tobi M, Ravid Z, et al: Increased $(2'-5')$-oligo-a synthetase activity in patients with prolonged illness associated with serological evidence of persistent Epstein-barr virus infection. Lancet 1:744, 1982.

102. Lusso P, Salahuddin SZ, Ablashi DV, et al: Diverse tropism of HBLV (human herpesvirus 6). Lancet 2(8561):743, 1987.

103. Glaser R, Kiecolt-Glaser JK: Stress-associated immune modulation: Relevance to viral infections and chronic fatigue syndrome. American Journal of Medicine 105(3A):35S-42S, 1998.

104. Ogawa M, Nishiura T, Yoshimura M, Horikawa Y, Yoshida H, Okajima Y, Matsumura I, Ishikawa J, Nakao H, Tomiyama Y, Kanayama Y, Kanakura Y, Matsu-zawa Y: Decreased nitric oxide-mediated natural killer cell activation in chronic fatigue syndrome. European Journal of Clinical Investigation 28(11):937-943, 1998.

105. See DM, Tilles JG: Alpha-interferon treatment of patients with chronic fatigue syndrome. Immunological Investigations 25(1-2):153-164, 1996.

106. Aoki T, Usada Y, Miyakoshi H: A novel immunodeficiency: Low NK syndrome (LNKS). Jap J Med 3212:14-17, 1985.

107. Miyakoshi H, Aoki T, Mizukoshi: Acting mechaanisms of Lentinan in humans. II. Enhancement of non-specific cell-mediated cytotoxicity as an interferon induced response. Int J Immunopharmacol 6:373-379, 1984.

108. Prieto J, Subira ML, Castilla A, et al: Naloxone-reversible monocyte dysfunction in patients with chronic fatigue syndrome. Scand J Immunol 30:13-20, 1989.

109. Gupta S, Aggarwal S, See D, Starr A: Cytokine production by adherent and non-adherent mononuclear cells in chronic fatigue syndrome. Journal of Psychiatric Research 31(1):149-156, 1997.

110. Conti F, Magrini L, Priori R, Valesini G, Bonini S: Eosinophil cationic protein serum levels and allergy in chronic fatigue syndrome. Allergy 51(2):124-127, 1996.

111. Steinberg P, Pheley A, Peterson PK: Influence of immediate hypersensitivity skin reaction on delayed reactions in patients with chronic fatigue syndrome. Journal of Allergy & Clinical Immunology 98(6 Pt 1):1126-1128, 1996.

112. Steinberg P, McNutt BE, Marshall P, Schenck C, Lurie N, Pheley A, Peterson PK: Double-blind placebo-controlled study of the efficacy of oral terfenadine in the treatment of chronic fatigue syndrome. Journal of Allergy & Clinical Immunology 97(1 Pt 1):119-126, 1996.

113. Baraniuk JN, Clauw D, MacDowell-Carneiro AL, Bellanti J, Pandiri P, Foong S, Ali M: IgE concentrations in chronic fatigue syndrome. Journal of Chronic Fatigue Syndrome 4(1):13-22, 1998.

114. Baraniuk JN, Clauw DJ, Gaumond E: Rhinitis symptoms in chronic fatigue syndrome. Annals of Allergy, Asthma, & Immunology 81(4):359-65, 1998.

115. Borish L, Schmaling K, DiClementi JD, Streib J, Negri J, Jones JF: Chronic fatigue syndrome: Identification of distinct subgroups on the basis of allergy and psychologic variables. Journal of Allergy & Clinical Immunology 102(2):222-230, 1998.

116. Borok G: Chronic fatigue syndrome: An atopic state. Journal of Chronic Fatigue Syndrome 4(3):39-58, 1998.

117. Vollmer-Conna U, Lloyd A, Hickie I, Wakefield D: Chronic fatigue syndrome: An immunological perspective. Australian & New Zealand Journal of Psychiatry 32(4):523-527, 1998.

118. Sheng WS, Hu S, Lamkin A, Peterson PK, Chao CC: Susceptibility to immunologically mediated fatigue in C57BL/6 versus Balb/c mice. Clinical Immunology & Immunopathology 81(2):161-167, 1996.

119. Rook GA, Zumla A: Gulf War syndrome: Is it due to a systemic shift in cytokine balance towards a Th2 profile? Lancet 349(9068):1831-1833, 1997.

120. Vojdani A, Lapp CW: Interferon-induced proteins are elevated in blood samples of patients with chemically or virally induced chronic fatigue syndrome. Immunopharm Immunotoxicol 21(2):175-202, 1999.

121. Klimas NG, Fletcher MA: Alteration of type 1/type 2 cytokine pattern following adoptive immunotherapy of patients with chronic fatigue syndrome (CFS) using autologous *ex vivo* expanded lymph node cells. Abstract, II International Conf. CFS, Brussels, 1999.

122. Dinarello CA: Interleukin-1 and interleukin-1 antagonism. Blood 77(8): 1627-1652, 1991.

123. Platanias LC, Vogelzang NJ: Interleukin-1: Biology, pathophysiology, and clinical prospects. Am J Med 89:621-629, 1990.

124. Patarca R, Lugtendorf S, Antoni M, Klimas NG, Fletcher MA: Dysregulated expression of tumor necrosis factor in the chronic fatigue immune dysfunction syndrome: Interrelations with cellular sources and patterns of soluble immune mediator expression. Clinical Infectious Diseases 18:S147-S153, 1994.

125. Linde A, Andersson B, Svenson SB, Ahrne H, Carlsson M, Forsberg P, Hugo H, Karstop A, Lenkei R, Lindwall A, et al: Serum levels of lymphokines and soluble cellular receptors in primary EBV infection and in patients with chronic fatigue syndrome. J Inf Dis 165:994-1000, 1992.

126. Rasmussen AK, Nielsen AH, Andersen V, Barington T, Bendtzen K, Hansen MB, Nielsen L, Pederson BK, Wiik A: Chronic fatigue syndrome–a controlled cross sectional study. J Rheumatol 21(8):1527-1531, 1994.

127. Morte S, Castilla A, Civeira MP, Serrano M, Prieto J: Production of interleukin-1 by peripheral blood mononuclear cells in patients with chronic fatigue syndrome. J. Infect Dis 159:362, 1989.

128. Straus SE, Dale JK, Peter JB, Dinarello CA: Circulating lymphokine levels in the chronic fatigue syndrome. J Inf Dis 160(6):1085-1086, 1989.

129. Arnason BGW: Nervous system–immune system communication. Rev Infect Dis 13(1):S134-S137, 1991.

130. Berkenbosch F, J Van Oers, A Del Rey, et al: Corticotropin-releasing factor-producing neurons in the RT activated by interleukin-1. Science 238:524-526, 1987.

131. Besedovsky H, Del Rey A, Sorkin E, et al: Immunoregulatory feedback between interleukin-1 and glucocorticoid hormones. Science 1986; 233:652-654, 1986.

132. Sapolsky R, Rivier C, Yamamoto G, et al: Interleukin-1 stimulates the secretion of hypothalamic corticotropin-releasing factor. Science 233:522-524, 1987.

133. Bernton EW, Beach J, Holaday JW, et al: Release of multiple hormones by a direct action of interleukin-1 on pituitary cells. Science 238:519-521, 1987.

134. Rettori V, Gimeno MF, Karara A, et al: Interleukin 1a inhibits protaglandin E_2 release to suppress pulsatile release of luteinizing hormone but not follicle-stimulating hormone. Proc Natl Acad Sci USA 88:2763-2767, 1991.

135. Shoham S, Davenne D, Cady AB, et al: Recombinant tumor necrosis factor and interleukin 1 enhance slow-wave sleep. Am J Physiol 253:R142-R149, 1987.

136. Holmes GP, Kaplan JE, Gantz NM, et al: Chronic fatigue syndrome: A working cased definition. Ann Intern Med 108:387-389, 1988.

137. Moldovsky H: Nonrestorative sleep and symptoms after a febrile illness in patients with fibrosis and chronic fatigue syndrome. J Rheumatol 16(19):150-153, 1989.

138. Van Eldik LJ, Zimmer DB: Secretion of S-100 from rat C6 glioma cells. Brain Res 436:367-370, 1987.

139. Griffin WST, Stanley LC, Ling C, et al.: Brain interleukin 1 and S-100 immunoreactivity are elevated in Down's syndrome and Alzheimer's disease. Proc Natl Acad Sci USA 86:7611-7615, 1989.

140. Dejana E, Brenario F, Erroi A, et al: Modulation of endothelial cell function by different molecular species of interleukin-1. Blood 69:635-699, 1987.

141. Caverzasio J, Rizzoli R, Dayer JM: Interleukin-1 decreases renal sodium reabsorption: Possible mechanisms of endotoxin-induced natriuresis. Am J Physiol 252:943-6, 1987.

142. Gulick T, Chung MK, Pieper SJ, et al: Interleukin-1 and tumor necrosis factor inhibit cardiac myocyte beta-adrenergic responsiveness. Proc Natl Acad Sci USA 86:6753-6757, 1989.

143. Cannon JG, Angel JB, Abad LW, Vannier E, Mileno MD, Fagioli L, Wolff SM, Komaroff AL: Interleukin-1 beta, interleukin-1 receptor antagonist, and soluble interleukin-1 receptor type II secretion in chronic fatigue syndrome. Journal of Clinical Immunology 17(3):253-261, 1997.

144. Beutler B, Cerami A: Cachectin (tumor necrosis factor). A macrophage hormone governing cellular metabolism and inflammatory response. Endocr Rev 9:57-66, 1988.

145. Kriegler M, Perez C, DeFay, et al: A novel form of TNF-cachectin in a cell surface cytotoxic transmembrane protein: ramifications for the complex physiology of TNF. Cell 53:45-53, 1988.

146. Wilt SG, Milward E, Zhou JM, et al.: *In vitro* evidence for a dual role of tumor necrosis factor in human immunodeficiency virus type 1 encephalopathy. Ann Neurol 37:381-394, 1995.

147. Dreisbach AW, Hendrickson T, Beezhold D, Riesenberg LA, Sklar AH: Elevated levels of tumor necrosis factor alpha in postdialysis fatigue. International Journal of Artificial Organs 21(2):83-86, 1998.

148. Dinarello C: Interleukin-1 and tumor necrosis factor: Effector cytokines in autoimmune diseases. Seminars Immunol 4(3):133-145, 1992.

149. Watson J, Mochizuki D: Interleukin-2: a class of T cell growth factor. Immunol Rev 51:257-278, 1980.

150. Fletcher M, Goldstein AL: Recent advances in the understanding of the biochemistry and clinical pharmacology of interelukin-2. Lymphokine Res 1:45-57, 1987.

151. Morgan DA, Ruscetti FW, Gallo RC: Selective *in vitro* growth of T lymphocytes from normal human bone marrows. Science 193:1007-1008, 1976.

152. Malkovsky M, Loveland B, Noth M, et al: Recombinant interleukin-2 directly augments the cytotoxicity of human monocytes. Nature 325:262-265, 1987.

153. Tsudo M, Ichiyama T, Uchino H: Expression of Tac antigen on activated normal human B cells. J Exp Med 160:612-617, 1984.

154. Cheney PR, Dorman SE, Bell DS: Interleukin-2 and the chronic fatigue syndrome. Ann Intern Med 110(4):321, 1989.

155. Cohen N, Stempel C, Colombe B, et al: Soluble interleukin-2 receptor: detection and potential role in organ transplantation. Clinical Immunology Newsletter 10(12):175, 1990.

156. Pui CH: Serum interleukin-2 receptor: clinical and biological implications. Leukemia 3(5):323-327, 1989.

157. Paul WE, Ohara J: B-cell stimulatory factor-1/interleukin-4. Annu Rev Immunol 5:429-459, 1987.

158. Kuehn R, Rajewsky K, Mueller W: Generation and analysis of interlekin-4 deficient mice. Science 254:713-716, 1991.

159. Chao CC, Gallagher M, Phair J, Peterson PK: Serum neopterin and interleukin-6 levels in chronic fatigue syndrome. J Infect Dis 162:1412-1413, 1990.

160. Chao CC, Janoff EN, Hu S, Thomas K, Gallagher M, Tsang M, Peterson PK: Altered cytokine release in peripheral blood mononuclear cell cultures from patients with the chronic fatigue syndrome. Cytokine 3:292-298, 1991.

161. Mizel SB: The interleukins. FASEB J 3:2379-2388, 1989.

162. Van Snick J: Interleukin-6: an overview. Ann Rev Immunol 8:253-278, 1990.

163. Penttila IA, Harris RJ, Storm P, Haynes D, Worswick DA, Marmion BP: Cytokine dysregulation in the post-Q-fever syndrome. QJM 91(8):549-560, 1998.

164. Lloyd A, Hanna DA, Wakefield D: Interferon and myalgic encephalomyelitis. Lancet 1:471, 1988.

165. Ho-Yen DO, Carrington D, Armstrong AA: Myalgic encephalomyelitis and alpha-interferon. Lancet 1:125, 1988.

166. Dalakas MC, Mock V, Hawkins MJ: Fatigue: Definitions, mechanisms, and paradigms for study. Seminars in Oncology 1998; 25(1 Suppl 1):48-53, 1998.

167. Jones TH, Wadler S, Hupart KH: Endocrine-mediated mechanisms of fatigue during treatment with interferon-alpha. Seminars in Oncology 25(1 Suppl 1): 54-63, 1998.

168. Pavol MA, Meyers CA, Rexer JL, et al.: Pattern of neurobehavioral deficits with interferon alpha tehrapy for leukemia. Neurology 45:947-950, 1995.

169. Davis JM, Weaver JA, Kohut ML, Colbert LH, Ghaffar A, Mayer EP: Immune system activation and fatigue during treadmill running: Role of interferon. Medicine & Science in Sports & Exercise 30(6):863-868, 1998.

170. Zlotnick A, Shimonkewitz P, Gefter ML, et al: Characterization of the gamma interferon-mediated induction of antigen-presenting ability in P388D cells. J Immunol 131:2814-2820, 1983.

171. Targan S, Stebbing N: *In vitro* interactions of purified cloned human interferons on NK cells: enhanced activation. J Immunol 129:934-935, 1982.

172. Knop J, Stremer R, Nauman C, et al: Interferon inhibits the suppressor T cell response of delayed hypersensitivity. Nature 296:757-759, 1982.

173. Bennett AL, Chao CC, Hu S, Buchwald D, Fagioli LR, Schur PH, Peterson PK, Komaroff AL: Elevation of bioactive transforming growth factor-beta in serum from patients with chronic fatigue syndrome. Journal of Clinical Immunology 17(2):160-166, 1997.

174. Bagasra O, Fitzharis JW, Bagasra TT: Neopterin: an early marker of development of pre-AIDS conditions in HIV-seropositive individuals. Clinical Immunology Newsletter 9:197-199, 1988.

175. Patarca R: Pteridines and neuroimmune function and pathology. Journal of Chronic Fatigue Syndrome 3(1):69-86, 1997.

176. Fuchs D, Muur C, Reibnegger G, Weiss G, Werner ER, Werner-Felmayer G, Wachter H: Nitric oxide synthase and antimicrobial armature of human macrophages. J Inf Dis 169:224, 1994.

177. Fuchs D, Baier-Bitterlich G, Wachter H: Nitric oxide and AIDS dementia. New Eng J Med 333(8):521-522, 1995.

178. Baier-Bitterlich G, Fuchs D, Murr C, Reibnegger G, Werner Felmayer G, Sgonc R, Böck G, Dierich MP, Wachter H: Effect of neopterin and 7,8-dihydroneopterin on tumor necrosis factor-alpha induced programmed cell death. FEBS Lett 364:234-238, 1995.

179. Lutgendorf S, Antoni MH, Ironson G, Fletcher MA, Penendo F, Van Riel F, Baum A, Schneiderman N, Klimas N: Physical symptoms of chronic fatigue syndrome are exacerbated by the stress of Hurricane Andrew. Psychosomatic Med 57:310-323, 1995.

180. Fuchs D, Moller AA, Reibnegger G, et al: Decreased serum tryptophan in patients with HIV-1 infection correlates with increased serum neopterin and with neurologic/psychiatric symptoms. J AIDS 3:873-876, 1990.

181. Iwagaki H, Hizuta A, Tanaka N, Orita K: Decreased serum tryptophan in patients with cancer cachexia correlates with increased serum neopterin. Immunological Investigations 24(3):467-478, 1995.

182. Heyes MP, Saito K, Milstein S, Schiff SJ: Quinolinic acid in tumors, hemorrhage and bacterial infections of the central nervous system in children. J Neurol Sci 133(1-2):112-118, 1995.

183. Saito K: Biochemical studies on AIDS dementia complex–possible contribution of quinolinic acid during brain damage. Rinsho Byori-Jap J Clin Pathol 43(9):891-901, 1995.

184. Shaskan EG, Brew BJ, Rosenblum M, Thompson RM, Price RW: Increased neopterin levels in brains of patients with human immunodeficiency virus type 1 infection. J Neurochem 59(4):1541-1546, 1992.

185. Andondonskaja-Renz B, Zeitler H: Pteridines in plasma and in cells of peripheral blood tumor patients. *In* Biochemical and clinical aspects of pteridines, Pfeiderer W, Wachter H, Curtius HC (eds.). Berlin-New York, Walter de Gruyter, 1984, pp. 295-311.

186. Sonnerborg A, Saaf J, Alexius B et al: Quantitative detection of brain aberrations in human immunodeficiency virus type 1-infected individuals by magnetic resonance imaging. J Inf Dis 162:1245-1251, 1990.

187. Buchwald D, Cheney PR, Peterson DL, Henry B, et al: Chronic illness characterized by fatigue, neurologic and immunologic disorders and active human herpesvirus 6 type infection. Ann Int Med 116:103-113, 1992.

188. Hamblin TJ, Hussain J, Akbar AN, et al: Immunological reason for chronic ill health after infectious mononucleosis. BMJ 287:85-88, 1983.

189. Tosato G, Straus S, Henle W, et al: Characteristic T cell dysfunction in patients with chronic active Epstein-Barr virus infection (chronic infectious mononucleosis). J Immunol 134:3082-3088, 1985.

190. Hilgers A, Frank J: Chronic fatigue syndrome: Evaluation of a 30-criteria-score and correlation with immune activation. Journal of Chronic Fatigue Syndrome 2(4):35-47, 1996.

191. Read R, Spickett G, Harvey J, et al: IgG1 subclass deficiency in patients with chronic fatigue syndrome. lancet 1:241-242, 1988.

192. Roubalova K, Roubal J, Skopovy P, et al: Antibody response to Epstein-Barr virus antigens in patients with chronic viral infection. J Med Viol 25:115-122, 1988

193. Salit IE: Sporadic postinfectious neuromyasthenia. Can Med Assoc J 133: 659-663, 1985.

194. Wakefield D, Lloyd A, Brockman A: Immunoglobulin subclass abnormalities in patients with chronic fatigue syndrome. J Pediatr Infect Dis 9(8):S50-S53, 1990.

195. Komaroff AL, Geiger AM, Wormsley S: IgG subclass deficiencies in chronic fatigue syndrome. Lancet 1:1288-1289, 1988.

196. Lloyd A, Hickie I, Wakefield D, et al: A double-blind, placebo-controlled trial of intravenous immunoglobulin therapy in patients with chronic fatigue syndrome. Am J Med 89:561-568, 1990.

197. Peterson PK, Shepard J, Macres M, et al: A controlled trial of intravenous immunoglobulin G in chronic fatigue syndrome. Am J Med 89:554-560, 1990.

198. Rowe KS: Double-blind randomized controlled trial to assess the efficacy of intravenous gammaglobulin for the management of chronic fatigue syndrome in adolescents. Journal of Psychiatric Research 31(1):133-147, 1997.

199. Straus SE: Intravenous immunoglobulin treatment for the chronic fatigue syndrome. Am J Med 89:551-553, 1990.

200. Vollmer-Conna U, Hickie I, Hadzi-Pavlovic D, Tymms K, Wakefield D, Dwyer J, Lloyd A: Intravenous immunoglobulin is ineffective in the treatment of patients with chronic fatigue syndrome. American Journal of Medicine 103(1):38-43, 1997.

201. Bennett AL, Fagioli LR, Schur PH, Schacterle RS, Komaroff AL: Immunoglobulin subclass levels in chronic fatigue syndrome. Journal of Clinical Immunology 16(6):315-320, 1996.

202. Konstantinov K, von Mikecz A, Buchwald D, Jones J, Gerace L, Tan EM: Autoantibodies to nuclear antigens in chronic fatigue syndrome. Journal of Clinical Investigation 98(8):1888-1896, 1996.

203. Poteliakhoff A: Fatigue syndromes and the aetiology of autoimmune disease. Journal of Chronic Fatigue Syndrome 4(4):31-50 1998.

204. von Mikecz A, Konstantinov K, Buchwald DS, Gerace L, Tan EM: High frequency of autoantibodies in patients with chronic fatigue syndrome. Arthritis & Rheumatism 40(2):295-305, 1997.

205. Keller RH, Lane JL, Klimas N, Reiter WM, Fletcher MA, van Riel F, Morgan R: Association between HLA class II antigens and the chronic fatigue immune dysfunction syndrome. Clin Inf Dis 18(Suppl 1):S154-S156, 1994.

206. Kaslow JE, Rucker L, Onishi R: Liver extract-folic acid-cyanocobalamin vs. placebo for chronic fatigue syndrome. Arch Intern Med 149:2501-2503, 1989.

207. Bates DW, Buchwald D, Lee J, Kith P, Doolittle T, Rutherford C, Churchill WH, Schur PH, Werner M, Wybenga D, et al: Clinical laboratory test findings in patients with chronic fatigue syndrome. Arch of Intern Med 155:97-103, 1995.

208. Nishikai M, Kosaka S: Incidence of antinuclear antibodies in Japanese patients with chronic fatigue syndrome. Arthritis & Rheumatism 40(11):2095-2097, 1997.

209. Weinstein L: Thyroiditis and "chronic infectious mononucleosis." N. Engl J Med 317:1225-1226, 1987.

210. Plioplys AV: Antimuscle and anti-CNS circulating antibodies in chronic fatigue syndrome. Neurology 48(6):1717-1719, 1997.

211. Cohen S, Tyrrell DA, Smith AP: Psychological stress and susceptibility to the common cold. N Eng J Med 325(9):606-612, 1991.

212. Glaser R, Rabin B, Chesney M, Cohen S, Natelson B: Stress-associated immune modulation: implications for infectious diseases? JAMA 281(24):2268-2270, 1999.

CLINICAL REPORTS

The Biorhythm of Fatigue in Chronic Fatigue Syndrome

J. Cabane
M. C. Renaud
K. P. Tiev

SUMMARY. Evidence is provided for a rhythmic interpretation of fatigue in CFS. *[Article copies available for a fee from The Haworth Document Delivery Service: 1-800-342-9678. E-mail address: <getinfo@haworthpressinc. com> Website: <http://www.haworthpressinc.com>]*

KEYWORDS. Biorhythm, chronic fatigue syndrome

Chronic fatigue syndrome (CFS) is a complex disease characterized by a dramatic lack of energy during months in previously healthy adults. The pathophysiology remains an enigma (1) since all known pathogens have been searched for unsuccessfully. According to a popular hypothesis, a central nervous system anomaly could be the cause. Hence, one of the synonyms of CFS (popular in the UK) is myalgic encephalo-

J. Cabane, M. C. Renaud, and K. P. Tiev are affiliated with the Service de Médecine Interne (pavillon de l'horloge 2), Hôpital Saint-Antoine, 184 Faubourg Saint-Antoine, 75571 Paris cedex 12, France.

Address correspondence to: Pr. J. Cabane at the above address (E-mail: jean. cabane@sat-ap-hop-paris.fr).

[Haworth co-indexing entry note]: "The Biorhythm of Fatigue in Chronic Fatigue Syndrome." Cabane, J., M. C. Renaud, and K. P. Tiev. Co-published simultaneously in *Journal of Chronic Fatigue Syndrome* (The Haworth Medical Press, an imprint of The Haworth Press, Inc.) Vol. 6, No. 3/4, 2000, pp. 109-116; and: *Chronic Fatigue Syndrome: Critical Reviews and Clinical Advances* (ed: Kenny De Meirleir, and Roberto Patarca-Montero) The Haworth Medical Press, an imprint of The Haworth Press, Inc., 2000, pp. 109-116. Single or multiple copies of this article are available for a fee from The Haworth Document Delivery Service [1-800-342-9678, 9:00 a.m. - 5:00 p.m. (EST). E-mail address: getinfo@haworthpressinc.com].

myelitis. Indeed, abnormalities have been described by some but not all authors in CFS patients in the temperature (2,3), sleep (4), melatonin (5,6), cortisol (7,8), heart rate variability (9), blood pressure (10), electro-encephalographic waves (11). Moreover, symptoms resembling those of CFS are frequently attributed to changes in the work schedule (12). In addition, fatigue is abundantly described as a consequence of jet lag.

In fact, the symptoms of CFS and chiefly the fatigue itself could vary. Among the number of patients followed at the Saint-Antoine unit, many tell that the course of CFS seems an irregular one, with periods of exacerbation and amelioration; however, according to the available literature concerning CFS, the question remains open as to whether or not fatigue, energy and mood fluctuate over the short- or the long-term (13-16). On the other hand, it is known that CFS is a spontaneously curable disease, and that towards the end fatigue becomes intermittent, the proportion of "fatigued" days decreasing progressively from 7 a week to 6/7 or 4/7, then 3/7, and so on. Thus, we started a prospective study to confirm that there exists a biorhythm of fatigue in CFS.

SUBJECTS AND METHODS

We sent a letter to 49 patients suffering from CFS fulfilling the international diagnostic criteria (1) and followed at the Saint-Antoine internal medicine center, asking them if they would report about their fatigue and evaluate it prospectively over a year. Ten patients (one American and nine French) agreed. They were first asked to answer a 20-item questionnaire about fatigue adapted in French from the MFI-20, a validated fatigue scale (17-19). The answers were converted in fatigue scores by the investigator on a scale from 1 to 5.

Second, they were asked to put on longitudinal scales the fatigue periods they felt prospectively: we chose to stratify them in two levels: moderate fatigue periods (defined as the periods where the activity and perceived energy levels are reduced from 30% to 50%) and severe fatigue periods (defined as the periods where the activity and perceived energy levels are reduced from 50% to 100%).

RESULTS

Fatigue Scores

The fatigue scores according to the adapted version of MFI-20 were computed and grouped 5 by 5 in 4 fatigue subgroups after Smets (17).

The mean fatigue scores were never less than 2/5; the fatigue subgroups scored more for physical (15, 2/25) and general fatigue (14, 7/25) than for either mental fatigue (10, 1/25) or diminished motivation (8, 1/25). The activity score fell in between the two (12, 2/25). We interpreted those results as showing that CFS patients are more handicapped from reduced physical capabilities than from mental inhibition.

Fatigue Biorhythm

Among the 10 patients, none had permanent fatigue. On the contrary, all described fluctuations in their CFS. One filled the questionnaire twice in order to show the difference between the "fatigue" periods and the "non-fatigue" ones (Figure 1).

FIGURE 1. Biorhythm of fatigue in an individual (Subject Fay): The same scale adapted MFI-20 was used both times, when the subject felt good ("Fay . . well") or fatigued (Fay . . bad). The clear bars show the data on good days and the dark ones on fatigued days.

Left part of the figure: individual items (range of each item: 0 to 5). Each individual item of the measuring tool scored answers to standardized questions about fatigue with scores between 1 and 5, 5 being the maximal fatigue score.

Right part of the figure: The scores were grouped 5 by 5 to give scores of general fatigue, physical fatigue, reduced motivation, mental fatigue and activity score.

The difference on the scale between "well" and "bad" days is visually obvious, but the score of the mental fatigue (as seen in the last clear bar) remained quite high even the "well," i.e., the non-fatigued days.

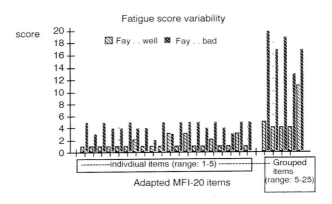

Timescale: 24 Hour

All subjects except one had more than one period of fatigue during the 24 hour period. There were few differences between weekend days and the other days. Two patients had only fatigue attacks during the day, and the majority had fatigue attacks during the night too (Figure 2), indicating that they were feeling fatigue even during sleep.

Timescale: Week

Five patients had no fluctuations during the week days. One felt a permanent fatigue and some fatigue peaks on Tuesdays and Wednesdays as well as Saturdays and Sundays. The four others had a clear weekly rhythm of fatigue, either once or twice a week (Figure 3).

FIGURE 2. Fluctuation of fatigue in CFS during the 24 hours (horizontal lines) of a representative work day (bars over the lines) and weekend day (bars under the lines). Only one patient (L) had a clear difference between workdays and weekend days. The majority of patients suffered from peaks of fatigue many times over the 24 hour period, and one (Ga) had a round-the-clock (albeit fluctuant) fatigue.

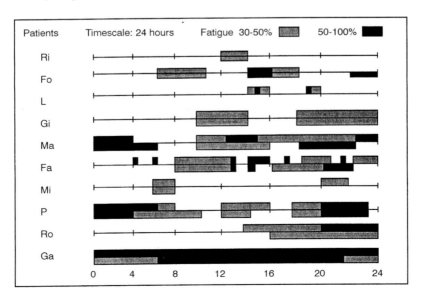

FIGURE 3. Variations in the fatigue according to the days in the week. Five patients had no variations. Among the 5 others, 2 had single weekly period of fatigue involving respectively one and four days, 2 had a biweekly pattern and 1 a permanent one with peaks of fatigue three times a week.

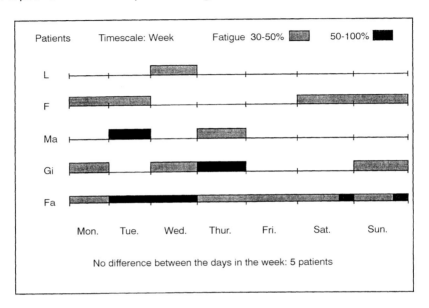

Timescale: Month

Five patients had no variations during the month and one had very little. Four had one, three, four or more fatigue peaks during a representative month (Figure 4).

Timescale: Year

Three patients had perannual fatigue and seven had variations in their fatigue over the year: 3 had one peaks, 2 had two peaks, 1 had four peaks and 1 a very irregular fatigue with a one-month remission (Figure 5).

DISCUSSION

We observed great differences between patients in this year-long study. This alone would justify the debate concerning the existence of

FIGURE 4. Variations in the fatigue among 5 patients with CFS over a representative month. One patient had a once-a-month pattern, another a permanent-with-two-peaks pattern. The others exhibited multiple monthly peaks of fatigue, giving patterns of fatigue on the basis of three, four or even more (subject Fa described his own as "machine-gun fatigue").

Five patients stated that there were no significant variations of their fatigue on a monthly basis.

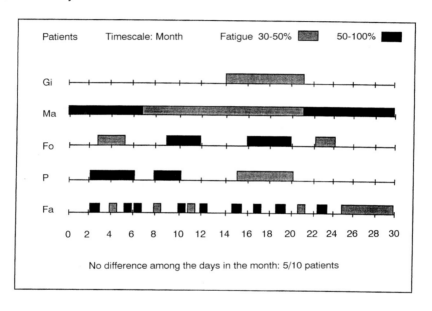

the fluctuating biorhythm and the variation of CFS symptoms in the available literature.

However, when examining the results of this selected population, either over the short-, medium- or long-term, the evidence is overwhelmingly in favor of a rhythmic interpretation of fatigue in CFS.

Whatever cause or causes are to be attributed to the CFS, they must take into account this peculiar pattern of fluctuation. Whatever the cause of CFS, it should injure the body structures involved in the biorhythm control, which leads us to hypothesize that the midbrain be involved. On the other hand, in the future research on CFS, it would be possible to use the CFS biorhythm to select among the multiple possible etiologies those fluctuating synchronously with the fatigue as the most plausible ones.

FIGURE 5. Variations of the fatigue level over the year among 10 patients with CFS. Three patients show a once-a-year pattern, 2 a twice-a-year one, 1 a seasonal pattern and 1 a throughout-the-year fatigue with a one month remission.
Three patients had no significant variation of their fatigue over the year.

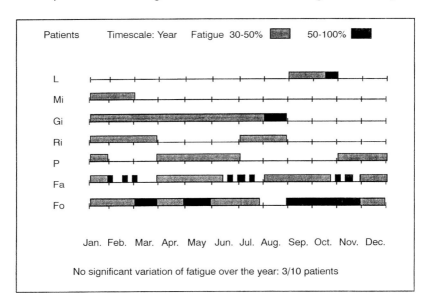

REFERENCES

1. Lloyd AR : Chronic fatigue and chronic fatigue syndrome: shifting boundaries and attributions. Am J Med 1998;105(3A): 7S-10S.

2. Camus F, Henzel D, Janowski M, Raguin G, Leport C, Vilde JL: Unexplained fever and chronic fatigue: abnormal circadian temperature pattern. Eur J Med 1992;1(1):30-6.

3. Hamilos DL, Nutter D, Gershtenson J, Redmond DP, Clementi JD, Schmaling KB, Make BJ, Jones JF: Core body temperature is normal in chronic fatigue syndrome. Biol Psychiatry 1998;43(4):293-302.

4. Moldofsky H: Sleep, neuroimmune and neuroendocrine functions in fibromyalgia and chronic fatigue syndrome. Adv Neuroimmunol 1995;5(1):39-56.

5. Williams G, Pirmohamed J, Minors D, Waterhouse J, Buchan I, Arendt J, Edwards RH : Dissociation of body-core temperature and melatonin secretion circadian rhythms in patients with chronic fatigue syndrome. Clin Physiol 1996;16(4):327-37.

6. Wikner J, Hirsch U, Wetterberg L, Rojdmark S : Fibromyalgia–a syndrome associated with decreased nocturnal melatonin secretion. Clin Endocrinol 1998;49(2):179-83.

7. Wood B, Wessely S, Papadopoulos A, Poon L, Checkley S: Salivary cortisol profiles in chronic fatigue syndrome. Neuropsychobiology 1998;37(1):1-4.

8. Strickland P, Morriss R, Wearden A, Deakin B: A comparison of salivary cortisol in chronic fatigue syndrome, community depression and healthy controls. J Affect Disord 1998;47(1-3):191-4.

9. Martinez-Lavin M, Hermosillo AG, Rosas M, Soto ME: Circadian studies of autonomic nervous balance in patients with fibromyalgia: a heart rate variability analysis. Arthritis Rheum 1998;41(11):1966-71.

10. van de Luit L, van der Meulen J, Cleophas TJ, Zwinderman AH: Amplified amplitudes of circadian rhythms and nighttime hypotension in patients with chronic fatigue syndrome: improvement by inopamil but not by melatonin. Angiology 1998;49(11):903-8.

11. MacFarlane JG, Shahal B, Mously C, Moldofsky H: Periodic K-alpha sleep EEG activity and periodic sleep movements during sleep: comparison of clinical features and sleep parameters. Sleep 1996;19(3):200-4.

12. Leese G, Chattington P, Fraser W, Vora J, Edwards R, Williams G: Short-term night-shift working mimics the pituitary-adrenocortical dysfunction in chronic fatigue syndrome. J Clin Endocrinol Metab 1996;81(5):1867-70.

13. Wood C, Magnello ME, Sharpe MC: Fluctuations in perceived energy and mood among patients with chronic fatigue syndrome. J R Soc Med 1992;85(4):195-8.

14. Zubieta JK, Engleberg NC, Yargic LI, Pande AC, Demitrac MA: Seasonal symptom variation in patients with chronic fatigue: comparison with major mood disorders. J Psychiatr Res 1994;28(1):13-22.

15. Garcia-Borreguero D, Dale JK, Rosenthal NE, Chiara A, O'Fallon A, Bartko JJ, Straus SE: Lack of seasonal variation of symptoms in patients with chronic fatigue syndrome. Psychiatr Res 1998;77(2):71-7.

16. Terman M, Levine SM, Terman JS, Doherty S: Chronic fatigue syndrome and seasonal affective disorder: comorbidity, diagnostic overlap, and implications for the treatment. Am J Med 1998;105(3A):115S-124S.

17. Smets EM, Garssen B, Bonke B, De Haes JC: The Multidimensonal Fatigue Inventory (MFI) psychometric qualities of an instrument to assess fatigue. J Psychom Res 1995;39(3):315-25.

18. Smets EM, Garssen B, De Haes JC: Application of the multidimensonal fatigue inventory (MFI-20) in cancer patients receiving radiotherapy. Br J Cancer 1996;73(2)241-5.

19. Schneider RA: Reliability and validity of the Multidimensonal Fatigue Inventory (MFI-20) and the Rhoten Fatigue Scale among rural cancer outpatients. Cancer Nurs 1998;21(5):370-3.

Divalent Cations, Hormones, Psyche and Soma: Four Case Reports

A. D. Höck, MD

SUMMARY. Objectives: The steroid hormone, vitamin D and the peptide hormone, parathormone are reported to influence not only bone metabolism, but also other metabolic and nervous, cardiovascular and immune functions, and mood. Regular actions of these hormones depend highly on intracellular magnesium content. Although symptoms are recognized, they usually are not correlated to these hormones. Foregoing case studies have revealed that vitamin D and/or parathormone disorders are common causes of CFS-fibromyalgia like symptoms.

Methods: Four patients with chronic fatigue-like symptoms and vitamin D (25OHD3) and parathormone (PTH intact) disorders are illustrated to demonstrate conflicting laboratory results. Patients were treated with 5,000 to 10,000 IU cholecalciferol, plus multiminerals and trace elements. Clinical outcome was assessed and treatment difficulties are reported.

Results: Diagnostic pitfalls are shown. Vitamin D and parathormone disorders are not completely detectable by calcium and phosphate screening. In 2 of this 4 demonstrated cases treatable diagnosis would have been missed without endocrinological screening. In the case of undetected long-standing disorder of these hormones, intracellular mineral derangement follows, thus inducing vitamin D resistance and parathormone ineffectiveness which makes therapy difficult. Combining vitamin D therapy with multiminerals possibly may overcome these obstacles.

A. D. Höck is in Practice of Internal Medicine and Psychotherapy, Hohenstaufen-ring 53, 50674 Köln, Germany, Europe.

[Haworth co-indexing entry note]: "Divalent Cations, Hormones, Psyche and Soma: Four Case Reports." Höck, A. D. Co-published simultaneously in *Journal of Chronic Fatigue Syndrome* (The Haworth Medical Press, an imprint of The Haworth Press, Inc.) Vol. 6, No. 3/4, 2000, pp. 117-131; and: *Chronic Fatigue Syndrome: Critical Reviews and Clinical Advances* (ed: Kenny De Meirleir, and Roberto Patarca-Montero) The Haworth Medical Press, an imprint of The Haworth Press, Inc., 2000, pp. 117-131. Single or multiple copies of this article are available for a fee from The Haworth Document Delivery Service [1-800-342-9678, 9:00 a.m. - 5:00 p.m. (EST). E-mail address: getinfo@haworthpressinc.com].

Conclusions: Vitamin D and parathormone disturbance should not be overlooked in chronic fatigue. Appropriate therapy is easy, inexpensive and harmless. Early diagnosis and treatment might be essential to avoid chronic fatigue syndrome. The complexity of diagnosis, therapy and scientific background may lead to a new understanding of "psychosomatic" disease. The relation between intracellular minerals, trace elements, cellular energy supply and responsible hormones should become clearer. *[Article copies available for a fee from The Haworth Document Delivery Service: 1-800-342-9678. E-mail address: <getinfo@haworthpressinc.com> Website: <http://www.haworthpressinc.com>]*

KEYWORDS. Divalent cations, vitamin D, parathormone, energy supply, hormone resistance, psychotropism of light induced hormones

BACKGROUND

Hypo- and hyperparathyroidism and vitamin D deficiency induce overlapping clinical signs. Hypoparathyroidism is associated with behavioral abnormalities, depression, psychosis, neural excitability, tetany, epilepsy, gastrointestinal and immunological dysfunction, tissue calcification, and premature arteriosclerosis (1). Normocalcemic hypoparathyroidism has been described (2). Hyperparathyroidism must be suspected when lethargy, fatigue, renal stones, constipation and/or other gastrointestinal irritation, bone pains and premature arteriosclerosis dominate the clinical picture (3). Vitamin D deficiency leads to irritability, nervousness, cerebral dysfunction, tetany, epilepsy (4), immune dysfunction (5,6), metabolic syndrome with hypertonus and diabetes (7). Magnesium deficiency induces reversible failure to secrete parathormone (8), thus leading to ineffective activation of vitamin D.

Numerous receptor binding sites for 1,25-dihydrocholecalciferol $[1,25(OH)_2D3]$, present in a wide range of different cell types, puts the calcium dogma of vitamin D in question (9). Influence on mood, possibly induced by serotonergic effects, is found by self reports of volunteers (10). The optimal ranges of 25-hydroxyvitamin D (25OHD3) levels and optimal substitution doses are not yet definitely defined (11-13).

METHODS

In foregoing studies, patients with fatigue of so-called unknown origin, i.e., with normal physical and routine laboratory results, but self reports of weakness, pains, functional disorder and intellectual impairment, according to chronic fatigue and chronic fatigue syndrome diagnostic criteria, were screened with respect to parathormone intact (PTH intact) and vitamin D (25OHD3) levels. In the case of pathological results, they were treated with doses of cholecalciferol according to the rickets prophylactics of childhood, but adjusted to weight and surface of adults. These doses were found most efficaceous by dose response studies in the years 1993 and 1994 (14). In some cases, vitamin D resistance became apparent, despite these higher doses of vitamin D substitution. Since January 1997, a mixture of minerals and trace elements, and since January 1999, additional calcium substitution in a dose from 500 to 2000 mg was added to influence resistant cases.

Four most extraordinary and striking cases were elected and are presented here to demonstrate the puzzling complexity of possible laboratory results, and the overall difficulties of diagnostic interpretation. In all cases, the first diagnosis and treatment option were revised later on.

	Case 1: B. A. 16.06.48, female	Case 2: L. I. 03.10.52, female	Case 3: B. J. 22.03.67, male	Case 4: Sch. M. 23.07.68, female
Clinical signs:	depression, fatigue, sleeping disorder, difficulty of concentrating, thinking and remembering, hair loss, diarrhea, drug rash, cold sweats	depression, fatigue, nervousness, back pain, sweats, trembling, epigastric pain, exertional dyspnea, overweight, periostitis, vitiligo	weakness, fatigue, myalgia, arthralgia, headaches, difficulty of concentrating, learning, thinking and remembering	chronic fatigue, but working; bone pain, myalgia, arthralgia, nausea, alcohol intolerance, exertional sweats, face flush, menometrorrhagia, easy bruising
routine laboratory results	Ca 2.3 mmol/L, Ph 1.2 mmol/L, Mg 0.85 mmol/L	Ca 2.98 mmol/L, Ph 0.5 mmol/L, Ca in urine 11.5 mmol/day, c-AMP 20 nmol (normal)	Ca 2.3 mmol/L, Ph 0.88 mmol/L, Mg 0.80 mmol/L, c-AMP 28 nmol (slightly elevated)	Ca 2.7 mmol/L, Ph 1.2 mmol/L
endocrinologic laboratory results	25OHD3 4 ng/ml PTH 112 pg/ml, ferritin 33 ng/ml	25OHD3 no data, PTH 155 pg/ml, ferritin 96 ng/ml	25OHD3 35 ng/ml, PTH 323 pg/ml, ferritin 25 ng/ml	25OHD3 7 ng/ml, PTH 3.3 pg/ml, ferritin 11 ng/ml
descriptive diagnosis	depression	secondary depression	CFS	somatoform disorder
first diagnosis (year of diagnosis marked)	1991, depression	1991, somatoform depression due to primary hyperparathyroidism	1997, CFS-like disease due to pseudohypoparathyroidism	1994, somatoform disorder due to hypoparathyroidism and vitamin D deficiency

	Case 1: B. A. 16.06.48, female	Case 2: L. I. 03.10.52, female	Case 3: B. J. 22.03.67, male	Case 4: Sch. M. 23.07.68, female
initial therapy	psychotherapy	parathroidectomy with implantation of a graft in the left forearm, dehydrotachysterol (AT 10)	cholecalciferol 5,000 IU/d, magnesium	cholecalciferol 10,000 IU/d, magnesium
first clinical outcome	deterioration	long-standing postoperative graft failure with hypo-parathyroidism, later on panic attacks	no response	partial response
revised diagnosis	vitamin D deficiency, secondary hyper-parathyroidism, secondary somatoform disorder (CFS)	postoperative hypopara-thyroidism, graft failure due to mineral deficits	hidden vitamin D deficiency? chronic mineral deficits with ineffective PTH?	hypopara-thyroidism and vitamin D deficiency due to long-standing mineral deficits following chronic vitamin D deficiency
revised therapy	cholecalciferol 10,000 IU/d, magnesium, other minerals, calcium	initially: 2 mcg/d calcitriol, and magnesium, than: addition of 5,000 IU/d cholecalciferol, magnesium, other minerals, calcium	cholecalciferol 5,000 IU/d, magnesium, other minerals, calcium	cholecalciferol 10,000 IU/d, magnesium, other minerals, calcium
clinical outcome after revised therapy	improvement of depression, fatigue and cognitive deficits. But minor sleeping disorder and new bone pains	improvement of depression, fatigue and vegetative signs. But metabolic syndrome. Parathormone rise to low normal	improvement of fatigue and pains	improvement of fatigue, pains and nausea. But recurrent iron deficiency. New: hypertension, back and leg pains

Normal:
serum Ca 2.2-2.6 mmol/L, serum Ph 0.9-1.5 mmol/L, serum Mg 0.70-1.06 mmol/L, urine Calcium: 2.5-8 mmol/day, 25OHD3 normal 7-49 ng/ml, optimal 30-50 ng/ml, PTH intact 12-72 pg/ml, ferritin 35-266 ng/ml

CASE REPORTS IN DETAIL

Case 1: B. A., Female, Borne June 16, 1948

Clinical signs: After a viral infection and death of mother in 1989, depression, chronic fatigue, sleeping disorder. Ineffective psychotherapy from 1991-1994 because of depression. Deterioration of clinical status up to 1993. Suspicion of chronic fatigue syndrome led finally to the correct endocrinological diagnosis in 1993. Just before the beginning of treatment with vitamin D, clinical picture changed to impending psychosis. Diarrhea, difficulty concentrating and remembering, irritability, listlessness, inappropriate laughing and crying, diffuse hair loss, drug induced rash, cold sweats had evolved.

Laboratory results: serum Ca 2.3 mmol/L (2.2-2.6), PTH intact 112 pg/ml (12-72), 25OHD3 4 ng/ml, control 3 ng/ml (8.7-50), 1,25(OH)$_2$ D3 1342 pg/ml (16-43).

Endocrinological diagnosis: secondary hyperparathyroidism due to vitamin D deficiency, secondary depression and behavior disorder.

Treatment and follow-up: 10,000 IU (250 mcg) cholecalciferol/day. Immediate recovery from signs of impending psychosis, but persistence of diarrhea and almost total hair loss. Total relapse after switch to the usually recommended dose of 500 IU (12.5 mcg). Addition of magnesium led to disappearance of diarrhea, addition of phosphate and potassium, in 1996, to growing of new hairs. In 1997 level of 25OHD3, 111 ng/ml. Dose reduction to 5,000 IU/day (125 mcg), followed by arthralgias and bone pain, resembling fibromyalgia and vitamin D resistance. Treatment was accomplished with mineral, trace elements. Since February 1999 extra calcium doses were added.

Case 2: L.I., Female, Borne October 3, 1952

Clinical signs: Fatigue, nervousness, listlessness, depression, back pains, sweats, trembling, epigastric discomfort, exertional dyspnea, overweight, periostitis, vitiligo.

Laboratory results: Ca in serum 2.98 mmol/L (2.2-2.6), Phosphate in serum 0.5 mmol/L (0.9-1.5), PTH intact 155 pg/ml (12-72), Calcium in urine 11.5 mmol/day (2.5-8), C-AMP in urine 20 nmol (normal), 25OHD3 not measured.

Endocrinological diagnosis March 1991: Primary hyperparathyroidism with secondary depression.

Treatment and follow-up: April 1991 resection of all 4 parathyroids, transplantation of one piece in the forearm. Postoperative PTH intact < 1 pg/ml until January 1998. Postoperative diagnosis: Hypoparathyroidism due to parathyroidectomy, graft insufficiency.

Treatment with 2 mg AT 10[®] (dihydrotachysterol)/day. In 1995 sudden onset of tetany and panic attacks. Switch from dihydrotachysterol to Rocaltrol[®] (calcitriol) 2 mcg/day and substitution of minerals and trace elements. Panic attacks subsided not completely. However, cholecalciferol 5,000 IU/day (125 mcg), given additionally, induced complete remission of tetany and panic attacks. During following months stepwise reduction of calcitriol was possible. March 1998

PTH intact was raised to 14 pg/ml. Patient felt well, had no panic attacks, she was able to abandon calcitriol with a switch 10,000 IU cholecalciferol/day.

New revised diagnosis March 1989: Tertiary hyperparathyroidism before operation, maybe due to long-standing undiagnosed vitamin D deficiency. Postresectional hypoparathyroidism and graft insufficiency due to mineral and vitamin D deficiency.

Case 3: B. J., Male, Borne March 22, 1967

Clinical signs: Weakness, fatigue, myalgia, arthralgia, headache, difficulty concentrating, learning and remembering. Descriptive psychiatric diagnosis: chronic fatigue syndrome.

Laboratory results: Labor: Ca in serum 2.3 mmol/L (2.2-2.6), Ph 0.88 mmol/L, 25OHD3 35 ng/ml (8.7-50), PTH intact 323 pg/ml (by laboratory kit from Immulite), c-AMP 28 nmol (slightly elevated).

Endocrinological diagnosis August 1997: Pseudohypoparathyroidism. Differential diagnosis: Secondary hyperparathyroidism due to hidden vitamin D-deficiency.

Treatment and follow-up: 5,000 I.E. (125 mcg) cholecalciferol/day and magnesium. Laboratory from March 1998: 25OHD3 77 ng/ml, PTH intact 203 pg/ml (by Immulite), 56 pg/ml (by Nichols), but complaints persisted. Since March 1999, addition of calcium and slow improvement.

Secondary revised diagnosis: Hidden vitamin D deficiency, severe calcium deficiency and total body mineral loss, secondary hyperparathyroidism (falsely extremely elevated by Immulite kit). The correlation of 203 (Immulite) to 56 ng/ml (Nichols) respectively, means, that in either case, there must have been an elevation of PTH intact before treatment.

Case 4: SCH. M., Female, Borne July 23, 1968

Clinical signs: School difficulties since the age of 10. Small for age, underweight, chewing nails, excoriation of skin at fingertips and toes, nail grooves, deep longitudinal furrow of the tongue, hyperplasia of nasal conchae, deviation of nasal septum. Since years chronic fatigue. Fell asleep when sitting down at home, but working in a job. Diffuse pains in bones, muscles and joints. Nausea, intolerance of alcohol with sensations of being paralyzed, cold sensations in lower back, exertion-al sweats, face flush, goose skin, easy bruising, frequent nose bleed-ing, menometrorrhagia. Persistent iron deficiency, even after cessation of abnormal uterine blood loss by hormonal treatment.

Laboratory results: Ca in serum 2.7 mmol/L (2.2-2.6), phosphate in serum 1.2 mmol/L (0.8-1.5), PTH intact 3.3 pg/ml (12-72), 25OHD3 7 ng/ml (8.7-50).

Endocrinological diagnosis April 1994: Hypoparathyroidism and vitamin D deficiency, but paradoxically elevated calcium in serum.

Psychiatric diagnosis: Minimal mental retardation, mild compul-sive disorder, somatoform disorder secondary to maybe long-standing endocrine disorder? Differential diagnosis: neuro-ectodermal disorder as inborn error of metabolism?

Treatment and follow-up: 10,000 IU cholecalciferol/day (250 mcg) and magnesium. Intermittent relief of pains and fatigue. December 1997 25OHD3 94 ng/ml. After reduction to 5,000 IU/day (125 mcg) new pains and fatigue. Patient too poor to afford multiminerals and trace elements. Addition of calcium since January 1999. Persistent hypertonus, chronic recurrent iron deficiency when iron supplements are abandoned. Back, hip and leg pains due to abnormal position of vertebral column. Patient no longer able to do her job.

RESULTS

The presented cases showed a wide array of clinical conditions, resembling depression, somatoform disorder, chronic fatigue syn-drome, mental retardation, compulsive disorder, and inborn errors of metabolism, respectively. Individual complaints did not foresee exact laboratory data. Only in cases 2 and 4, serum calcium was elevated, and in case 2, phosphate diminished, thus pointing to an underlying endocrine disorder. In cases 1 and 3, diagnosis would have been missed totally.

Case 1 with its low normal serum calcium and phosphate levels demonstrates the typical case of secondary hyperparathyroidism, fol-lowing chronic vitamin D deficiency. Almost complete alopecia made pseudohypoparathyroidism with casual vitamin D deficiency a prob-able differential diagnosis of this case. Alopecia, fatigue, severe nerv-ousness and intellectual impairment reversed after treatment. Fibromyalgia-like complaints of bone pains and sleeping disorder, however, persist despite ongoing therapy, on to now.

A much more complex pattern is found in the other cases.

In case 2, initially typical signs of primary hyperparathyroidism prevailed, except for the nonelevated c-AMP. In 1991, the importance of investigating vitamin D level was not realized, thus not examined. After parathyroidectomy, it soon became clear, that forearm parathyroid graft function was ineffective. Under AT 10 treatment, serum calcium persisted at low normal levels, and tetany and panic attacks evolved. In suspicion of deranged calcium metabolism as a possible cause of psychiatric decompensation, a treatment switch to calcitriol and magnesium, finally combined with cholecalciferol, multiminerals and trace elements, was initiated. Cholecalciferol had proved good psychotropic results in foregoing case studies. In this case finally it could be used as the unique safe and unexpensive vitamin D substitution. Rising PTH intact after these switches correlated with disappearance of clinical signs. Growth and developing suppleness of the graft could be felt by finger print. The functional reserve of grafted parathyroid tissue seems remarkable, regaining endocrine activity after 7 years. However, metabolic syndrome with hypertension, as mentioned in literature, has meanwhile established. The effectiveness of additional calcium on metabolic syndrome has to be watched further on.

In case 3 the results showed a very high PTH intact level, done by the assay from Immulite, combined with a low normal calcium, on the one side, with optimal 25OHD3 level on the other side, according to either pseudohypo-parathyroidism or possibly hidden vitamin D deficiency. PTH intact by Nichols would have shown some elevation, but not thus extreme. At that time I was not aware, that there might be different kit results. Family history showed no suspicious cases of hyperparathyroidism and parents screening proved to be normal. During treatment parathormone fell to 203 pg/ml (Immulite), to 56 pg/ml respectively (Nichols). But no clinical response could be seen, unless calcium was added.

In case 4 inadequate low parathormone and very low levels of 25OHD3, despite high serum calcium and normal phosphate, were found. This case is the most opposite to described endocrinologic science. Poverty might have caused chronic vitamin D and secondary chronic mineral deficiency. Though bone pains soon abated and fatigue diminished after treatment initiation, the early onset of hypertension and the chronic iron deficiency is striking, later on followed by new bone pains, maybe due to skeletal imbalance.

In conclusion of these cases we have to learn that contradictory routine and endocrinological labaratory results put established and well-known endocrinological dogmata in question. Secretion of parathormone seems not in every case be triggered by magnesium exclusively, as described in literature, but might be optimized by substituting all main intracellular minerals, like magnesium, potassium, calcium, phosphate, complemented by trace elements, an observation maybe not realized in the past. Though vitamin D supplements were much higher than usually recommended, never hypercalcemia or renal calculi could be observed, even after addition of calcium up to 2,000 mg/day. Given single components alone did not reach the good results of combined treatment. Remarkably low treatment costs may be an obstacle to get pharmaceutical research supports for broader studies.

DISCUSSION

The symptom triads fatigue, functional disorder and pains should lead to a prompt search for the possible and not infrequent disturbances of divalent cations by investigating both vitamin D and parathormone. Mere screening for serum calcium and phosphate would overlook these treatable diseases in most cases, as seen in foregoing studies (not published). Low calcium, low phosphate and high parathormone levels are rare, low or low normal vitamin D and/or low parathormone intact levels are not rare. Even inadequate high parathormone values must be considered, dependent on the used assay kit. Metabolic syndrome as a very common condition might be a late somatic consequence of missed diagnosis. Serum phosphate is highly dependent on feeding state and on day time hour (15). Only ionized calcium, not serum total calcium, is a regulating substrate of parathormone (16).

In order to understand why derangements of these hormones mimic chronic fatigue syndrome or fibromyalgia, we should look at 7 important items, so at parathormone and vitamin D, their functional interdependence with other hormones, their possible relation to stress response, the role of calcium and magnesium and the interdependence of intracellular minerals with any other cellular component.

1. The peptide hormone parathormone is a multihormone with mul-

tiple active centers influencing mineral metabolism, cell function, and vitamin D metabolism. The carboxy-terminal center at amino acid 84 is said to regulate the transport of divalent cations. The amino-terminal center induces c-AMP as important second messenger and the vitamin D activating 1-α hydroxylase function (17).

2. The steroid hormone vitamin D behaves even more multifunctionally. Vitamin D metabolites interact directly with cell membranes and influence membrane fluidity. By this nongenomic pathway, ion channels and other membrane proteins get influenced (18). $1,25(OH)_2D3$ induces by its genomic pathways the synthesis of calbindin 9, a calcium and phosphate transporting, and of calbindin 28 KD, a calcium binding EF-hand protein, the latter functionally comparable to calmodulin. $1,25(OH)_2D3$ induces the synthesis of Ca-ATPase, 1-α-hydroxylase, 24-hydroxylase and alkaline phosphatase and alters protein synthesis of other proteins, e.g., proto-oncogene products, protein kinase C, polyamine synthesis enzymes, tissue specific proteins, calmodulin acceptor proteins, creatine kinase, other metabolic enzymes and hormone agonist receptors (19,20). As a not well understood effect until now, $1,25(OH)_2D3$ influences cell differentiation, proliferation and cell cycle regulation (21-23).

3. $1,25(OH)_2D3$ interact with other hormones, modulating and fine-tuning their actions through endocrine, paracrine, and autocrine functional properties. But not only $1,25 (OH)_2 D3$ seems to have important functions. The non-calciotropic 24,25-dihydroxychole-calciferol $[24,25(OH)_2D3]$ might be a very important metabolite as well and seems to counterbalance some actions of $1,25(OH)_2D3$ (24,25). Inborn modifications of vitamin receptor might explain needs for higher substitution doses than usually recommended, though results are very controversially discussed (26). Modulation of receptor abundance is another point of concern (27). Further minor inborn polymorphism of transcriptional machinery, even intracellular mineral imbalance by itself, might explain different function of transcriptional machinery as well (28). Vitamin D deficiency or resistance and/or parathormone deficiency or resistance induce secondary immunological and endocrine events. Vitamin D normally downregulates TH1 as well as TH2 answers, whilst optimizing macrophage differentiation and actions, thus contributing to an efficient immunological competence (29).

4. Parathormone and vitamin D have to be added to the family of stress response modulating hormones. Stress regulation is dependent

on further light-dependent psychotropic hormones. The so-called "zeitgeber" (30) is influenced directly by light, but might interact with light-dependent hormones. Parathormone is indirectly light dependent, since it's genetically influenced by $1,25(OH)_2D3$ (31). Light related mitigation of stress response are already described with respect to MSH (32) and melatonin (33). Mallette elucidates that the prohormone proopio-melano-corticotropin (POMC) is enzymatically cleaved to ACTH and melanocyte stimulating hormone (α-MSH), both cleavage products showing striking homology in some parts of their sequence with parathormone. ACTH, α-MSH and parathormone can bind partly to the other's membrane receptors. Prepro-PTH, the prehormone of parathormone, and POMC are discussed to have a common genetic origin. The fundamental importance of parathormone in psycho-neuro-immunologic interplay becomes evident.

5. Parathormone and vitamin D act both on divalent cations and also on the important anion phosphate. Long-standing suboptimal or clearly reduced vitamin D levels induce intracellular disturbance of mineral metabolism, in particular calcium, magnesium and phosphate deficiency. These deficiencies, by themselves, lead to resistance of both hormones, thus introducing a vicious cycle (34-37). Calcium is important for tissue as a structurally stabilizing factor, functionally important for cellular signal transduction by being a second messenger, binds to the large family of intracellular EF-hand proteins thus multiplying and ramifying calcium signals, binds to cell membrane adjacent proteins interacting in cellular locomotion, cellular adhesion and fusion mechanisms and is important for nuclear, RES and mitochondrial function. Calcium is able to bind tightly up to 12 oxygen atoms, for instance to negative glutamate or aspartate or neutral glutamine and asparagine residues or carbonyl groups. Thus, calcium helps, in the tissue, to hold structural protein array, reduces hydrogen and water content of tissues, helps intracellularly with protein function to become strongly determinated and quick enough and with pH keeping in a physiological range. Magnesium is able to bind to oxygen as well, but 1,000 times weaker than calcium. Magnesium forms symmetrical protein cores, calcium is able to form asymmetrical and much greater cores, enabling multiple and widespread enzymatic interactions (38).

Considering all these data we must learn that calcium deficits must be linked to cellular, nuclear, RES and mitochondrial dysfunction, as well as to intercellular and cell-tissue cross-talk dysfunction due to impaired signal transduction and protein synthesis, acidosis, deprived energy stores and impaired tissue protein conformation (39,40).

6. Magnesium by itself is important for cellular energy balance. Three important ATP-driven ion pumps need magnesium as a cofactor to work efficiently (41). That means that magnesium deficiency results in cellular potassium leak due to compromised K-Na-exchanger, diminished ATP-production due to the compromised H-pump, and raised free intracellular calcium due to compromised Ca-ATPases. Raised intracellular free calcium as second messenger then influences the other main intracellular messenger pathways, for instance c-AMP. Considering these interactions, once more, the strong correlation between mineral metabolism, functional performance and energy stores becomes clearer.

7. As a highly interdependent functional system, the main intracellular cations potassium and magnesium, the phosphate stores in the form of ATP, free intracellular calcium and the bound calcium stores, trace elements, vitamins, proteins and all other cellular compounds are proportionally and structurally bound and interrelated. Therefore, any isolated intracellular derangement, not only mineral deficits but also toxic influences or oxidative stress, drives the cell to find a new balance, in reducing cell structure by means of down-regulating protein synthesis by elevated free intracellular calcium (42). All these conditions override cellular "well-being."

Common causes of "fatigue," like for instance, lack of sunlight, or calcium and phosphate depletion after ongoing lack of sunlight, or loss of minerals by excessive exercise, or common nutritional deficiencies like magnesium deficiency, due to artificial fertilizer, or iron deficiency following menometrorrhagia, or inborn low detoxification or redox capacity might be some of the everyday conditions to acquire chronic fatigue syndrome. The common general pathway of all these conditions seems to be raised intracellular free calcium, reduced intracellular and organelle calcium stores, deprivation of cellular energy production and protein catabolism, followed by cellular dysfunction and cell signal resistances. Pains might represent the biological signal of severe cellular and tissue distress.

A totally new and complex understanding of disease and its "psycho-somatic" human expression arises by considering newly detected insights of modern biochemistry and molecular biology.

REFERENCES

1. Sherwood LM, Santora II AC: Hypoparathyroid States in the Differential Diagnosis of Hypocalcemia. In: Bilezikian JP, ed. The Parathyroids, Basic and Clinical Concepts. New York, Raven Press, 1994: 747-52.

2. Potts, JT: Diseases of the Parathyroid Gland and Other Hyper- and Hypocalcemic Disorders. In: Fauci AS, ed. Harrisons's Principles of Internal Medicine, New York: MacGraw-Hill, Inc. 1998: 2227-47.

3. Bilezikian JP, Silverberg SJ, Gartenberg F, Kim TS, Jacobs TP, Siris ES, Shane E: Clinical Presentation of Primary Hyperparathyroidism. In: Bilezikian JP, ed. The Parathyroids, Basic and Clinical Concepts. New York, Raven Press, 1994: 457-69.

4. Carswell S: Vitamin D in the Nervous System: Actions and Therapeutic Potential. In: Feldman D, ed. Vitamin D, New York, Academic Press, 1997: 1197-1211.

5. Lemire J: The Role of Vitamin D_3 in Immunosuppression: Lessons from Autoimmunity and Transplantation. In: Feldman D, ed. Vitamin D, New York, Academic Press, 1997: 1167-81.

6. Hewison M, O'Riordan JLH: Immunomodulatory and Cell Differentiation Effects of Vitamin D. In: Feldman D, ed. Vitamin D, New York, Academic Press, 1997: 447-62.

7. Mathieu CH, Casteels K, Bouillon R: Vitamin D and Diabetes. In: Feldman D, ed. Vitamin D, New York, Academic Press, 1997: 1183-96.

8. Rude RK: Parathyroid Function in Magnesium Deficiency. In: Bilezikian JP, ed. The Parathyroids, Basic and Clinical Concepts. New York, Raven Press, 1994:829-42.

9. Stumpf WE: Vitamin D Sites and Mechanisms of Action: A Histochemical Perspective. Reflections on the Utility of Autoradiography and Cytopharmacology for Drug Targeting. Histochem Cell Biol, 1995; 104: 417-27.

10. Lansdowne ATG, Provost SC: Vitamin D enhances Mood in Healthy Subjects during Winter. Psychopharmacology. Springer Verlag 1998; 135: 319-23.

11. Thomas MK, et al.: Hypovitaminosis D in Medical Inpatients. N Engl J Med, 1998; 338: 777-83.

12. Utiger RD: The Need for More Vitamin D. N Engl J Med, 1998; 338: 828-9.

13. Vieth R: Vitamin D Supplementation, 25-Hydroxyvitamin D_3 Concentrations and Safety. Am J Clin Nutr 1999; 69: 842-56.

14. Höck AD: Fatigue and 25-Hydroxyvitamin D levels. JCFS, 1997; 3(3): 117-27.

15. Hruska K, Gupta A, Bonjour J, Caversazio J: Regulation of Phosphate Transport. In: Feldman D, ed. Vitamin D, New York, Academic Press, 1997: 499-519.

16. Brown EM: Homeostatic Mechanisms Regulating Extracellular and Intracellular Calcium Metabolism. In: Bilezikian JP, ed. The Parathyroids, Basic and Clinical Concepts. New York, Raven Press, 1994: 15-54.

17. Mallette LE: Parathyroid Hormone and Parathyroid Hormone-Related Protein as Polyhormones: Evolutionary Aspects and Nonclassical Actions. In: Bilezikian JP, ed. The Parathyroids, Basic and Clinical Concepts. New York, Raven Press, 1994: 171-184.

18. Norman AW: Rapid Biological Responses Mediated by 1α,25-Dihydroxyvitamin D3: A Case Study of Transcaltachia (Rapid Hormonal Stimulation of Intestinal Calcium Transport). In: Feldman D, ed. Vitamin D, New York, Academic Press, 1997: 233-56.

19. Holick MF: Noncalcemic Actions of 1,25-Dihydroxyvitamin D3 and Clinical Implications. In: Vitamin D. Physiology, Molecular Biology and Clinical Applications. Holick MF ed. Humana Press, Totowa, New Jersey. 1999; 207-16.

20. Walters MR: Other Vitamin D Target Tissues: Vitamin D Actions in Cardiovascular Tissue and Muscle, Endocrine and Reproductive Tissues, and Liver and Lung. In: Feldman D, ed. Vitamin D, New York, Academic Press, 1997: 463-82.

21. Boyan BD, Dean DD, Sylvia VL, Schwartz Z: Cartilage and Vitamin D: Genomic and Nongenomic Regulation by 1,25(OH)$_2$D$_3$ and 24,25(OH)$_2$D$_3$. In: Feldman D, ed. Vitamin D, New York, Academic Press, 1997: 395-421.

22. Thomasset M: Calbindin 9K. In: Feldman D, ed. Vitamin D, New York, Academic Press, 1997: 223-32.

23. Christakos S et al.: Calbindin D 28K. In: Feldman D, ed. Vitamin D, New York, Academic Press, 1997: 209-21.

24. Stumpf WE, Privette TE: Light, Vitamin D and Psychiatry. Psychopharmacology, 1989; 97: 285-94.

25. Hollis BW: Detection of Vitamin D and Its Major Metabolites. In: Feldman D, ed. Vitamin D, New York, Academic Press, 1997: 587-606.

26. Pike JW: The Vitamin D Receptor and Its Gene. In: Feldman D, ed. Vitamin D, New York, Academic Press, 1997: 105-25.

27. Krishnan V, Feldman D: Regulation of Vitamin D Receptor Abundance. In: Feldman D, ed. Vitamin D, New York, Academic Press, 1997: 179-200.

28. Issa LL et al.: Molecular Mechanism of Vitamin D Receptor Action. Inflamm Res 1998: 451-75

29. Adams JS: Extrarenal Production of Active Vitamin D Metabolites in Human Lymphoproliferative Diseases. In: Feldman D, ed. Vitamin D, New York, Academic Press, 1997: 903-21.

30. Stratakis CA, Chrousos GP: Neuroendocrinology and Pathophysiology of the Stress System. In: Chrousos GP, ed. Stress. Basic Mechanisms and Clinical Impactions. The New York Academy of Sciences, New York, 1995; 771: 1-18.

31. Silver J, Naveh-Many T: Vitamin D and the Parathyroid Gland. In: Feldman D, ed. Vitamin D, New York, Academic Press, 1997: 353-67.

32. Jegou S et al.: Regulation of α-Melanocyte-Stimulating Hormone Release from Hypothalamic Neurons. In: Chrousos GP, ed. Stress. Basic Mechanisms and Clinical Impactions. The New York Academy of Sciences, New York, 1995; 1: 260-78.

33. Brzezinski A: Melatonin in Humans. N Engl J Med 1997; 336: 186-95.

34. Carpenter TO: Disturbances of Vitamin D Metabolism During Clinical and Experimental Magnesium Deficiency. Magnesium Research 1988; 131-9.

35. Thacher TD et al.: A Comparison of Calcium, Vitamin D, or Both for Nutritional Rickets in Nigerian Children. N Engl J Med 1999; 341: 563-68.

36. Bishop N: Rickets Today—Children Still Need Milk and Sunshine. N Engl J Med 1999; 341: 602-3.

37. Drezner MK: Clinical Disorders of Phosphate Homeostasis. In: Feldman D, ed. Vitamin D, New York, Academic Press, 1997: 733-53.

38. Krebs J: Calcium Biochemistry. In: Meyers RA, ed. Encyclopedia of Molecular Biology and Molecular Medicine, Volume 1, Weinheim, New York, Basel, Cambridge, Tokyo 1996; 237-50.

39. Lehninger AL: Mitochondria and Calcium Ion Transport. Biochem J 1970, 119: 129-38.

40. Alberts B et al.: Cells in Their Social Context. In: Alberts B, ed. Molecular Biology of the Cell. Garland Publishing, Inc. New York 1994: 971-95.

41. Saeed MG et al.: Magnesium Deficiency: Pathophysiologic and Clinical Overview. Am J Kidney Dis, 1994; 24: 737-75234.

42. Vojdani A, Lapp W: The Relationship Between Chronic Fatigue Syndrome and Chemical Exposure. J Chron Fatigue Syndr, 1999; 5(3/4): 207-21.

Common Clinical and Biological Windows on CFS and Rickettsial Diseases

C. L. Jadin, MD, MBBCh

SUMMARY. From 1991, links between CFS and Rickettsial Diseases were uncovered because of their similar clinical presentation. Further research linked them even more. Five Rickettsia strains, suspected to be the cause, or an important factor in CFS, were identified by means of the Giroud Micro-Agglutination test and were widely found to be positive in patients' serum, diagnosed as suffering from CFS, Fibromyalgia, Rheumatoid Arthritis, Multiple Sclerosis, Depression, Psychosis, Heart Diseases, and Auto-Immune Diseases. This finding leads us to submit those originally differently diagnosed patients to the same tetracycline treatment. This proved to be a great success. The increasing number of patients gave us the opportunity to establish a biological checklist (regardless of the diversity of the pathology) of infections, organs' functions and auto-immune profile. We found the differences in positivity to depend on four factors: length of illness, virulence of germs, cohabitation of germs, and the state of the host immune system. These studies suggest that auto-immune diseases could have an infectious origin. Better knowledge and mastery of the co-factors would be determinant in speeding recovery. With this approach, CFS patients are being treated for the cause of their illness rather than symptomatically. *[Article copies available for a fee from The Haworth Document Delivery Service: 1-800-342-9678. E-mail address: <getinfo@haworthpressinc.com> Website: <http://www.haworthpressinc.com>]*

KEYWORDS. Intracellular organisms, clinical and biological changes, cellular anoxemia, CFS

C. L. Jadin, Postnet Suite 182, Private Bag X3, North Riding, 2162, Republic of South Africa (E-mail: gerinjadin@icon.co.za).

[Haworth co-indexing entry note]: "Common Clinical and Biological Windows on CFS and Rickettsial Diseases." Jadin, C. L. Co-published simultaneously in *Journal of Chronic Fatigue Syndrome* (The Haworth Medical Press, an imprint of The Haworth Press, Inc.) Vol. 6, No. 3/4, 2000, pp. 133-145; and: *Chronic Fatigue Syndrome: Critical Reviews and Clinical Advances* (ed: Kenny De Meirleir, and Roberto Patarca-Montero) The Haworth Medical Press, an imprint of The Haworth Press, Inc., 2000, pp. 133-145. Single or multiple copies of this article are available for a fee from The Haworth Document Delivery Service [1-800-342-9678, 9:00 a.m. - 5:00 p.m. (EST). E-mail address: getinfo@haworthpressinc.com].

133

Ceux auquels nous devons rendre compte de nos travaux, la societé, ne nous demandent pas tant de tracer des aperçus généraux que de trouver quelque chose qui soit pratique pour le diagnostique, la prévention et le traitement des maladies.

Charles Nicolle

INTRODUCTION

From 1991, links between CFS and chronic Rickettsial infection were uncovered, because of their similar constellation of symptoms (1). Further research in both fields linked them even more (2):

- CFS and Chronic Rickettsial Infection present with a similar symptomatology.
- CFS was first reported in Incline, Nevada in 1984 (3) and developed into epidemic proportions. Rocky Mountain Spotted Fever originated from the same place in 1916 (4). Drury described the spirochete *Borrelia duttoni*, in 1702 as causing the recurrent Malgache fever. In 1975, *Borrelia burgdorferi* was found in Connecticut, giving birth to a new name, Lyme Disease.
- A link has been established between CFS and Florence Nightingale (5) working surrounded by lice, fleas and ticks, during the Crimean war. Soldiers were presenting with epidemic typhus, the common disease of wars, regularly reported since the time of Hannibal up to modern times.
- Lymphocyte studies conducted on sheep with tick-borne diseases (6), CFS patients and patients with Q Fever endocarditis (14) are showing similar results.
- Coincidentally, the new name suggested in *Lancet* for CFS is PQFS (Post Q Fever Syndrome) (7) in April 1996 edition.
- The success rate of treating CFS patients with tetracyclines by Prof. J.B. Jadin, Prof. Legac, Prof. Giroud since 1963; Dr. Bottero since 1981, Dr. Tarbleton (8) since 1993, and myself since 1991 (9), shows a recovery rate of 84-96%.

MATERIALS AND METHODS

Almost all 3,600 patients presented with one common denominator: FATIGUE–often from a post infectious or post stress situation.

Table 1 is an analysis of 500 randomly selected patients previously diagnosed or treated for many other and various diseases, which never have been related before.

Secondly we therefore found the second common denominator: RICKETTSIAL INFECTION.

The examination opens *three windows:* the Symptomatic Window, the Clinical Window, and the Biological Window which are presented in Tables 2, 3, and 4. We find a positive Coombs test in two patients that were presenting with an acute condition (one Sjögren, one non-diagnosed). *These windows are generally applicable to all patients with FATIGUE regardless of the original diagnosis.*

DIAGNOSIS OF CHRONIC RICKETTSIAL INFECTION

Together with the Syptomatology, the clinical examination and our Biological checklist, Chronic Rickettsial Infection is established by the Micro-Agglutination test of Giroud-Jadin against the following five strains:

TABLE 1

ME, CFS, Fibromyalgia	320
Multiple Sclerosis	19
Epilepsy	4
Depression, Psychotic Disorders, Concentration Disorders in Children	40
Rheumatoid Arthritis	75
Scleroderma	2
Psoriatic Arthritis	4
Sjögren Syndrome	2
Crest Syndrome	1
Morphea	1
Valve replacement	3
High blood pressure	2
None	27

- *R. prowazeki:* the epidemic type of Typhus
- *R. mooseri*, which is endemic
- *R. conori*, which belongs to the spotted fever group
- *Coxiella burnetti*, which is well known as Q Fever. It has 2 phases; Phase II is pathogenic
- Neo Rickettsia Chlamydiae Q18 which falls into the Neo-Rickettsia group.

The antigens of those Rickettsiae are directly collected from the bowels of infected ticks and other arthropods, then mixed in a solution, injected into the peritoneal cavity of guinea pigs, mice, hamsters or rabbits or embryonated eggs to be cultivated (10).

Before releasing for testing, the solution is attenuated with formol.

The main source of antigens used in the MATG laboratory comes from Moscow. The Chlamydiae Q18, have been commercialised by the Mérieux Institute of Lyon. The Epidemic Typhus Antigens have been produced by the South African Institute for Medical Research.

Important Points

a. A high reading means a high serological level of antibodies–a negative reading in endemic areas reflects the poverty of the immune system (11).

b. Agglutination happens or does not–therefore there is no possibility of personal interpretation. Test quality depends on antigen quality (12).

c. Quality controls are done with:

   - Negative sera
   - Pure antigens, regularly checked to ensure the absence of auto-agglutination.

d. Variation of the curve of antibodies in time reveals the presence of active foci (11).

e. If doubtful or negative, in the presence significant symptomatology, the test should be repeated to follow the antibodies' curve.

f. Tests can give a negative reading if patients are treated with cortisone.

g. Positive tests can be found in people who display no symptoms (Giroud, Jadin [13]; 26% according to Drancourt and Levy [14]).

h. Comparative studies with the immunofluorescence test and the ELISA test performed by Prof. Jadin and a French Laboratory gave very similar results (15).
i. The BRUMPT prize of the Pasteur Institute of Paris was awarded to Prof. J.B. Jadin for this test in October 1997.
j. The test is currently done in the MATG laboratory in Johannesburg, South Africa upon request, for doctors in France, Italy, Germany, Belgium, Australia, South Africa and Zimbabwe.
k. The use of attenuated antigens is not accepted in the majority of laboratories because of the dangers they are said to present to the workers (16,17).

TREATMENT

Seven to 12 days a month of tetracyclines.

- On a *high dosage* with limitation: (18)
    - Safety (19,20)
    - Tolerance is attained with adjuvants like vitamin B co, *Acidobacillus*, and a gastric pump inhibitor
    - Herxheimer Reaction; which is a reactivation and/or exacerbation of old symptoms that occurs on antibiotherapy. Its presence has a very important diagnosis and prognosis value (11).
- The tetracyclines are *alternated* because we are dealing with:
    - Many strains of Rickettsiae (17)
    - And to avoid resistance (8,17)
- So we *combine* them with
    - Quinolones, • Macrolides, • Metronidazole, because Rickettsiae have a wide heterogenicity of susceptibility to different drugs (21)
- The treatment is *extended* due to:
    - Germ chronicity (10)
    - Multiple foci (10)
    - Inactive Rickettsiae, encapsulated and so protected from antibiotherapy (17)

- Each treatment stimulates the immune system by releasing Rickettsiae from the cell to the bloodstream, which will increase the production of antibodies (11)
- The *length* of the disease does not imply lengthy treatment
- *Antimalaria* are used to improve rheumatoid symptoms and rheumatoid biological findings (2)
- *Cortisone* is avoided as we are dealing with germs (15)
- *Exercise* is recommended because:

  - Rickettsiae are vascular diseases (11,14)
  - Rickettsiae like CO_2 atmosphere (22)
  - Rickettsiae like a low host metabolism (23)

- *Hot baths* are to assist in the elimination of toxins (17).

This treatment follows the French School and has been progressively honed through daily experience, trying to reach better efficiency and tolerance. It is never used intravenously (19). It has delivered very good results since 1991 (2,9). Through regular controls, clinical and biological, on patients undergoing treatment, and through questionnaires sent to a sample of 500 patients after treatment in 1996, no short- or long-term toxicity has been reported (2,21).

In 1995, a similar antibiotherapy was presented for Gulf War Illnesses (2), the important difference being the length of the treatment cycle and the specific rotation and combination of antibiotherapy.

RESULTS

Results are demonstrated by the clearing of the three windows (2,9) (Tables 2, 3, 4).

Symptoms are fading, activities increasing, from bedridden to exercise or back to work. From being treated with:

Painkillers,	
Anti-inflammatories	
Antidepressants	
Sedatives	to *NONE*
Shock therapy	
Cortisone	
Excessive vitamin and mineral supplements	

TABLE 2. Symptomatic Window

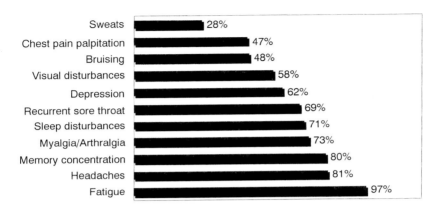

TABLE 3. Clinical Window

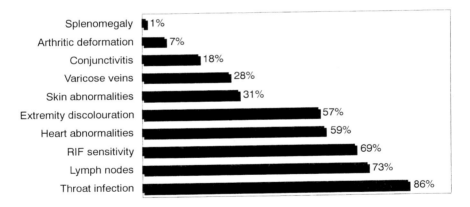

The *medical examination* improves or normalises.

- Brain scans improved in two MS patients.
- Fatty infiltration disappeared in liver scan (2 cases).
- EEG normalised in 3 epileptic patients (23).
- Ulcers healed in the morphea case (for whom a left leg amputation had been recommended).
- Rashes and eczema disappeared.
- Rheumatoid patients recover the use of their hands and feet.

TABLE 4. Biological Window

Test	Percentage
TFT	3%
KFT	8%
ESR	23%
FBC (abs monocytosis)	30%
Thyroid AB	39%
CRP, RF, ANF	48%
Iron	50%
Mycoplasma	62%
LFT	64%
Chlamydiae non spec	67%
Lympho study	71%
Rickettsial infection	87%

The *blood test* results improve or normalize.

Reinfection may obviously occur. Reactivation (called so rather than relapse) may also happen due to the interaction of bacteria, virus, stress, pollution, etc., causing the Rickettsiae, like many intracellular organisms, to change from dormant to active (24).

DISCUSSION

1. The above study shows an *infectious origin* of CFS-like diseases, sometimes simple (quick progress on treatment), sometimes complex (slow progress on treatment).

2. CFS can be linked to *Rickettsial-like diseases.* Two decades ago, Mycoplasma, Chlamydiae, Erlichioses were classified as sub groups of Rickettsiae (15,18). This is still in use in Russia (25), although those groups are today generally spread apart. Rickettsiae are found throughout the world, except in Antarctica, where they do not survive. In cold countries, there are as many germs, but less vectors and those vectors have less contact with humans (26).

3. Not only are Rickettsiae known to paralyse the macrophage population at sites, producing a monocytosis (49), but *due to their selective vascular affinity*, those germs might cause an amazing spectrum of diseases, according to the vessels they damage (28):

- CFS, fibromyalgia, where they cause a cellular anoxemia (2,9).
- Cardio-vascular diseases (11,15,18,29,30,31,32,33,34,35).
- Neurological diseases (from acute encephalitis to multiple sclerosis, epilepsy, etc.) (1,15,18,35).
- Abdominal diseases (appendicitis [12] and others).
- Ocular diseases (uveitis, retinal angiopathy, optic nevritis sometimes a long time after a general infection) (4,15).
- Auto-immune diseases (2,9,36).

Those diseases might evolve alone or in association, for example, Encephalomyocarditis described by Jadin (15).

4. The super-imposition of germs (viruses, bacteriae, parasites) on the immune system will lead to its bankruptcy (2,9,36), which will favor the multiplication of parasites, but *due to their obligated intracellular localization*, they will produce molecular changes, which will confuse the immune system and lead to *auto-immune diseases*. The confirmation of this affirmation lies in the 2 following facts:

   a. Thyroid Antibodies, Rheumatoid Factor, C Reactive Protein, Anti Nuclear Factor are usually (48%) in our study elevated, separated or together in patients serologically positive for Rickettsiae, Mycoplasma and Chlamydiae (Rheumatoid Factor 28%, C Reactive Protein 29%, AN, Anti Nuclear Factor 11.5%, Thyroid Antibodies 39%).
   b. The above blood tests often return to normal after Tetracycline pulse therapy, sometimes as early as after 6 months and remain normal (regular controls).

SUGGESTIONS FOR THE FUTURE

1. In the presence of CFS, Fibromyalgia, Auto-immune diseases, Heart diseases, MS, Depression, the screening for *Rickettsial-like infections* might be a valuable tool for treatment.
2. *Systematic Giemsa or Machiavello stain* of removed tissue (appendix, valves, vessels, peripheral glands, tonsils, spleen, brain tumours, placenta of aborted foetus) as done for Heartwater disease in cattle brains could improve diagnosis.

3. While waiting for a more practical test than the Micro-Aggluti-nation test of Giroud, the antigens should be commercialised and therefore be available to any laboratory in order to improve the diagnosis of Rickettsial diseases as a routine practice in the presence of *FATIGUE*.

4. Specific isolation and identification of Rickettsiae in different countries would lead to a world-wide comparative study of those microorganisms and a better understanding of their cycle, their virulence and their cohabitation. The implementation without delay of a global co-ordinated approach at this time is crucial to confine the germ and cure the disease.

5. Since *Chlamydiae* have been isolated in the cerebrospinal fluid of *MS* patients (Legac, Jadin, 1962 [4], 1986 [18], Sriram, Mitchell 1998 [37] and also in *cardiac valves,* Shor in RSA, 1992 [30]); equally since *Rickettsiae* have been isolated from Mitral and Aortic valves (Grist in Glasgow, 1963 [11], Dran-court in 1990 [14] and are known to cause *Endocarditis, Myo-carditis and Pericarditis* [1,11,13,18,21,28,29,31,38,39]), the use of *cortisone* depressing immune reaction should be re-stricted before infectious investigation.

6. Considering that *Cancer* consists of an altered cell population (40), could the *molecular changes* induced in the hosts' cells by an invading organism such as Rickettsiae be a simple switch of its mechanism (as suggested by Legac)? Cancer could then evolve independently masking the triggering mechanism.

7. Germs and their hosts are forming an *eco-system*. This is the most complex level of organisation in Nature, depending on cli-mate, water, nutrients, and energy. Due to the gap in our knowl-edge concerning basic parasite-host interaction (38), adminis-tration of *nutritional supplements and diet* are a hazardous guess, since it might *support the parasite rather than the host,* e.g., magnesium, glutamate, pyruvate are the principle energy-yielding substrate of Rickettsiae (11,41), ethanol kills Rickett-siae in vitro (5), folic acid supports some leukaemia cells.

8. The evolution of germs through *History* might lighten the co-factors necessary for the birth, the life and the death of diseases. To describe a *germ*, isolated, as a novelty is ignoring its impera-tive to *adapt* and *mutate* (42) in order to survive, so that it does not disappear like the Egyptian and Mayan civilizations. This

suggests that intracellular germs like Mycoplasma, Rickettsiae, Chlamydiae, Psittachosis, Erlichioses, Tularaemia and Brucellosis, having the same vector, could be mutants of the same germ and thus could need the same therapy.

9. To prevent the huge *economic* impact and further *complication* due to the chronicity of Rickettsial-like diseases, we emphasise *early diagnosis* and *treatment* or prevention of this condition.

10. Instead of producing *atoms* of research and discovery isolated in time and space, we stress the importance of linking our efforts world-wide between the past, present and future research.

REFERENCES

1. Jadin JG. Au Sujet des Maladies Rickettsiennes. *Annale de la Societé Belge de Medécine Tropicale* 1962; Vol 3: 321.

2. Jadin CL. The Rickettsial Approach of CFS. *CFS Manly Conference, Australia* February 1999.

3. Mauff G & Gon M. CFS in Incline Village. *SA Medical Journal* March 1991

4. Jadin JB. Origine des maladies Rickettsiennes. *Annale de la Societé Belge de Medécine Tropicale* 1953; Vol 3; pp. 1ff.

5. Hennessy T. CFS: May 12: F. Nightingale's Birthday; A Comprehensive Approach. *Annales Internationales de Medécine* 1994; 121; 953-959.

6. Woldehiwet Lymphomatic Subpopulations in Peripheral Blood of Sheep Experimentally infected with Tick-Borne Disease. *Research Vet. Scient.ist* July 1991.

7. Marmion BP, Shannon M. et al. Post Q Fever Syndrome. *Lancet* April 1996; Vol 347: 977-978.

8. Tarbleton P. "To Whom It May Concern." *Affidavit to the SA Medical Council* January 1995

9. Jadin CL. The Rickettsial Approach of CFS. *The Clinical and Scientific Basis of CFS.* T.K. Roberts ed. *University of Newcastle, Australia* 1998; 200-213.

10. Giroud P, Capponi M. Le Diagnostic des Rickettsioses. *Extrait du Traité de Biologie Appliqué* Paris: Librairie Maloine S.A., 1963.

11. Gear J, Monteiro Nicolau S, Bernard SG, Grist NR, Giroud P, MasBernard A. Roche A propos des Rickettsioses. *Bulletin Societé de Pathologie Exotique* 1963; 588-740.

12. Giroud P, Jadin J. Les Rickettsioses de nos Jours. *Extrait de Bulletin de L'Academie Nationale de Médecine* Vol 1; 58: N° 1.

13. Jadin J. Les Rickettsioses. Trent Ans après Charles Nicolle. *Academie Royale des Sciences d'Outre Mer* 1963; 6: 1128-1129.

14. Drancourt M & Levy MG. Rickettsial Infection. *8th Congress of the American Rickettsial Society* 1990.

15. Jadin J. Rickettsioses and Neurological Etiology *Acta Mediterranea di Patologia. Infectiva e Tropicale* 1987; 6: 213.

16. McDade JE. Rickettsiae. *Manual of Clinical Microbiology 5th Ed.* 1992; 1036 p.

17. Ormsbee JR. Rickettsiae. *Manual of Clinical Microbiology 4th Ed.* 1985; 845-855.

18. Aymard. Bourde. Giroud. Jadin. Legag. Bottero. *Clinique de la Résidence du Parc* 1986.

19. Bettina Schön Tetracycline in ME–Fad or Fact? *South African Medical Journal* 1992; 82.

20. Ives TJ, Manzewitsch P. *In vitro Susceptibilities of Rickettsiae.* University of NC, 1997: 578-582

21. Raoult D. Antibiotic Treatment of Rickettsioses, Recent Advances and Current Concepts. *European Journal of Epidemiology.* 1991; 7(3): 276-281.

22. Sande MA & Mandell GL. Antimicrobiological Agents Tetracyclines. In: *Pharmalogical Basis of Therapeutics* Goodman & Gilmans, 1991: 8th Ed.Vol 2.

23. Jadin CL. *EEG Report of 18 Year Old Epilectic* Pietermaritzburg February 1998.

24. Jadin JB. Relation entre Protozoaires, Virus et Bacteries. *Revue de la Association Belge des Laboratoire* 1984.

25. Timasheva OA. Rickettsiae. *Russian Journal of Microbiology, Epidemiology and Immunobiology* April 1998: Vol 2: 49-51.

26. Jadin JB. Persistance des Rickettsies. *Académie Royale des Science d'Outre-Mer* 1991.

27. Govan J, McFarlane I & Callander A. Monocytes. *Pathology Illustrated* 1981: 554.

28. Walter P. Infectious Diseases and Medical Microbiology. In: Braude, ed. *International Textbook of Medicine* 2nd Ed. P810-810 814

29. Brouqui Ph. et al. Chronic Q Fever. *Archive de. Internal Medicine* March 8 1993; 1: 642-648

30. Cho Chou Kuo, Shor et al. Demonstration of Chlamydiae Pneumonia in Artheroscllerotic Lesions of Coronary Arteries. *Department of Pathology SA.* April 1992

31. Jadin JB. Importation D'Oiseaux Exotiques et Neo-Rickettsies. *Bulletin Societé Pathologie Exotique* 1969

32. Penninger J. Chlamydia Protein Linked to Heart Disease. *Science Magazine* Feb 1999; 283.

33. Welsby P. Does Infection Cause Coronary Disease? *Update.* The City Hospital, Edinburgh, Nov. 1997: 15

34. Nuhlestein JB, Hammon EM, et al. Chlamydia and Artherosclerosis. *Journal of the American College of Cardiology.* June 1996: 27(7); 1555-61.

35. Carp RI. Multiple Sclerosis. *The Journal of Experimental Medicine* 1972; 136: 618.

36. Giroud P, & Jadin JB. Les Infections Superposées Sont à la Base des Faillites de L'Humanité. *Archive de L'. Institut Pasteur de Tunis.* 1986: Vol 63 97-99.

37. Sriram, Mitchel, Stratton. MS and Chlamydia Pneumoniae Infection of the CNS. *Department of Neurology Vanderbilt University Medicine Center, Nashville* Feb 1998: 571-2.

38. Philip RN. Historical Ruminations: Rickettsioses and the Rocky Mountain Laboratory. Preface. *Annals of New York Acadamy of Science* 1990; 1: pp. 1ff.

39. Telly BL et al. Minocycline in Rheumatoid Arthritis. *Annales of Internal Medicine* January 1995; 122(2): 81.

40. Howers A & Baylin SB. Biology of Human Neoplasia. *The Principle and Practice of Medicine* 21st Ed. 1984; Ch. 62, 607.

41. Brezinia R et al. Rickettsiae and Rickettsial Diseases. *Bulletin of the World Health Organization.* 1973; 49: 433-442.

42. Jadin JB. Evolution des Organismes Intracellulaires. *Archives de L'Institut Pasteur de Tunis* 1986: pp. 1ff.

Role of Rickettsiae and Chlamydiae in the Psychopathology of Chronic Fatigue Syndrome (CFS) Patients: A Diagnostic and Therapeutic Report

Philippe Bottero, MD

SUMMARY. Objective: To demonstrate the probable role of intracellular bacteria like Rickettsiae and Chlamydiae in the development of certain chronic psychopathological conditions and according to the efficiency of antibiotic regimes (cyclines and/or macrolides).

The letter aim is based on the fact that all the patients that I have seen since 1981 had a sera reaction positive for Rickettsiae and/or Chlamydiae using the micro-agglutination on blade technique of P. Giroud and M.L. Giroud (MAG) by Prof. J.B. Jadin of Antwerpen, Belgium with special antigens cultured on guinea pig lungs and chicken embryos.

Methods: This is an open study which began in 1981 in a private medical practice, not versus placebo; but with random choice. Treat-

Philippe Bottero is Faculté de Medecine, Paris, France, General Practitioner, and Member of International College of Rickettsiologists, 1987.

Address correspondence to: Philippe Bottero, Faculté de Medecine, Paris, France, 10 Avenue Henri Rochier 26110 Nyons, France (E-mail: p.botter@caramail.com).

The author thanks the French military doctor General P. Legac, and Professor Agrégé J. B. Jadin of Antwerp, Belgium who trained him in the field of chronic rickettsiae/chlamydiae diseases. He also thanks Ivor and Katerine Porter for translations, and Pascal Rolin for his help with the word-processor.

[Haworth co-indexing entry note]: "Role of Rickettsiae and Chlamydiae in the Psychopathology of Chronic Fatigue Syndrome (CFS) Patients: A Diagnostic and Therapeutic Report." Bottero, Philippe. Co-published simultaneously in *Journal of Chronic Fatigue Syndrome* (The Haworth Medical Press, an imprint of The Haworth Press, Inc.) Vol. 6, No. 3/4, 2000, pp. 147-161; and: *Chronic Fatigue Syndrome: Critical Reviews and Clinical Advances* (ed: Kenny De Meirleir, and Roberto Patarca-Montero) The Haworth Medical Press, an imprint of The Haworth Press, Inc., 2000, pp. 147-161. Single or multiple copies of this article are available for a fee from The Haworth Document Delivery Service [1-800-342-9678, 9:00 a.m. - 5:00 p.m. (EST). E-mail address: getinfo@haworthpressinc.com].

ment was for a minimum of six months (cyclines and/or macrolides together with vasodilatory medication; chloroquine; warm baths).

Group one: 98 CFS cases; women: 78, men: 20; for 67 cases, the ancientness of symptoms is more than 2 years.

Group two: 59 psycho-somatic cases; 5 schizophrenia; 3 borderline; 10 children with agressivity, excitement; 1 autistic child; 1 delirium with relapses.

Results: Group one: 79.5% good and very good results; 4.1% fairly good; 16.4% failed. Group two: 82.3% good and very good results; 2.5% fairly good; 15.2% failed.

Conclusion: This diagnostic and therapeutic study began in 1981.

All of the Dr. Bottero's therapeutic results are confirmed since 1991 by Dr. Cecile Jadin of Randburg (South Africa) for more than 3000 CFS and other psychopathological states (300): Sydney 98 CFS Conference, Australia.

We have shown that Rickettsiae and Chlamydiae are probably causative factors in many "psychopathologies." *[Article copies available for a fee from The Haworth Document Delivery Service: 1-800-342-9678. E-mail address: <getinfo@haworthpressinc.com> Website: <http://www.haworthpressinc.com>]*

KEYWORDS. *Rickettsia*, *Chlamydia*, antibiotics

INTRODUCTION

Rickettsiae and Chlamydiae are small gram negative bacteria. Rickettsiae are transmitted by the bite of ticks, lice, fleas, or, in certain special circumstances, by exposure to infected dust, cows, sheep, goats (*Coxiella burnetii*) and by drinking raw milk. Chlamydiae are transmitted by sexual contact (*Chlamydia trachomatis*), by exposure to cows, sheep, goats, pigeons, parrots, etc. (*Chlamydia psittaci*). The principal Rickettsiae and Chlamydiae in Europe are *R. conotii, R. prowazekii, R. mooserii, C. burnetii, Chlamydia trachomatis, C. pneumoniae, C. psittaci.*

Many writers, after Charles Nicolle (NL 19), have shown the clinical and epidemiological importance of the long survival of Rickettsiae in the reticular endothelial system and the walls of blood vessels. They are liable to be activated by an acute or hidden infection after delays of differing duration and are capable of initiating a chronic pathology. Professor Paul Giroud of the Pasteur Institute of the Academy of Medicine, the Army doctor Colonel P. Legac and Professor J.B. Jadin, previously of the School of Tropical Medicine, Antwerp, Belgium, have been central to this research.

Since World War II, many workers have reported that Rickettsiae and Chlamydiae are involved in chronic psychopathology and have noted concomitant vascular problems, both peripherical and central (LM 61, LM 62 and MAS 63). Others have shown Rickettsiae associated with the development of neurological illnesses (LM 61 and MAS 63).

During the International Conference on Rickettsiae in Palermo in 1987, we presented a paper (BOT 87), reporting 60 differing cases of psychopathology associated with Rickettsiae and Chlamydiae and circulatory and other problems. Also important are the endothelial and adventitial vascular tropism of Rickettsiae (Fraenkel's nodule) and their secretion of vasoconstrictive toxins (GW 58).

Diagnosis is confirmed by the laboratory testing of a blood serum sample using the micro-agglutination on blade technique of P. Giroud and M.L. Giroud (MAG) by Prof. Jadin of Antwerp, Belgium, with special antigens cultured on guinea pig lungs and chicken embryos. *R. conorii, R. mooserii and R. prowazekii* can present cross reactions.

In France, there are discrepancies between different laboratories, even when they use an identical method (IFI). Indeed, the value of the serologocal test seems to depend on the antigenic quality of the strains, which vary according to the conditions of their culture: for instance *C. burnettii* phase 1; phase 2.

Comment about Giroud test: (BOT 1987) numerous positive Giroud test have been confirmed by the IFI reaction both by Prof. Jadin and in a french laboratory and in ELISA on 28 sera.

A total of 22/22 were positive in MAG and 20/22 positive in IFI at low or medium levels (Lab Merieux, antigens cultured on cells). Twenty-eight sera positive in ELISA vis à vis *R. conorii* (Prof. J.B. Jadin strains) with presence of IgG in 81.5% of cases and presence of IgM in 82% of cases (Virology Department of C.H.U. of Grenoble France: Perron H. 1985).

On the other hand, all our cases have an important variation in the antibody titres from one examination to another. The Australian biologists B. Liedtke, B. Paspaliaris found in 1998 that 50% of 36 CFS sera have IgG antibodies against *C. burnetii* (27 kDa outer membrane protein) using an ELISA test. In my study in France, 55% of 70 CFS sera have antibodies against *C. burnetii* using the old P. Giroud serologic reaction. A recent study reported positive Q fever results in controls worldwide averaging around 8% (KKH93).

The central idea is the association with each Psychiatric diagnosis of symptoms of a vascular type both peripheral and/or central. Treatment of the patient is based on repeated courses of antibiotics (cyclines and/or macrolides) together with vasodilatory medication, chloroquine, and warm baths.

MATERIALS AND METHODS

This is an open study which began in 1981 in a private medical practice in France; not versus placebo, but with random choice. Treatment was for a minimum of six months (cyclines and/or macrolides together with vasodilatory medication, chloroquine, and warm baths).

Group One: 98 CFS Patients

The number of the most common individual symptoms are shown on Table 1 for 76 patients. Observed reactions, with the respective numbers of patients for each, are listed in Table 2 for 70 patients.

For 98 CFS

Women: 78   Men: 20

The ages of the group (Table 3):

- Less than 15 years: 0
- 15 to 30 years: 21
- 31 to 60 years: 69
- More than 60 years: 7
- Undetermined: 1

Treatment durations: Six months to over 6 years.

Ancientness of symptoms (Table 4):

- Less than 2 years: 9
- 2 to 5 years: 23

- More than 5 to 10 years: 19
- More than 10 to 20 years: 16
- More than 20 years: 9
- Undetermined: 22

TABLE 1. Number of the most common individual symptoms (for 76 patients)

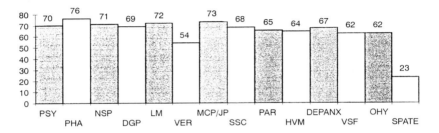

- Psychasthenia: PSY
- Physical asthemia: PHA
- Neuro-sensorial problems of a circulatory type: NSP
- Digestive problems: DGP
- Loss of memory: LM
- Vertigo: VER
- Muscular pain/Joint pain: MCP/JP

- Sensitivity to cold: SSC
- Paresthesis: PAR
- Headache/vascular migraine: HVM
- Depression/anxiety: DEPANX
- Vascular fragility: VSF
- Orthostatic hypotension: OHY
- Spasmophily tetany: SPATE

TABLE 2. Numbers of patients for each bacteria (for 70 patients)

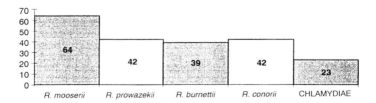

TABLE 3. Ages of the group

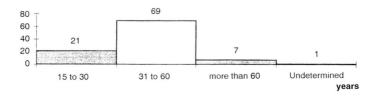

Results of the treatment (Table 5)

- Very good: 47 (47.9%), Good: 31 (31.6%), Total: 78 (79.5%)
- Fairly good: 4 (4.1%)
- Failed: 16 (16.4%)

Stop of treatment before 6 months for 16 patients (Table 6)

- Improved: 7
- Failed: 6
- Undetermined: 3

TABLE 4. Ancientness of symptoms

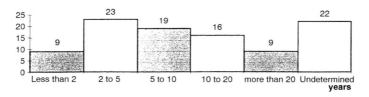

TABLE 5. Results of treatment

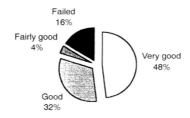

TABLE 6. Stop of treatment before 6 months (for 16 patients)

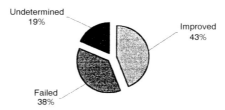

Because we know that 60% of CFS cure spontaneously before 2 years (Table 7), 67 cases have been isolated of which ancientness of symptoms are more than 2 years.

Result of treatment:

- Good and very good: 78%
- Fairly good: 5%
- Fail: 17%

Group Two

Seventy-nine psychopathological states (59 psycho-somatic; 5 schizophrenia; 3 border-line; 1 delirium with relapses; 10 children with agressivity, excitement; 1 autistic child).

Fifty-nine "psycho-somatic" cases associated with peripheral and central vascular problems; often with depression/anxiety sometimes with spasmophily/tetany and phobia/obsession symptoms (often improved).

Women: 33   Men: 26

Ages of the group:

- Less than 15 years: 4
- 15 to 30 years: 20
- 31 to 60 years: 29
- More than 60 years: 4
- Undetermined: 2

Ancientness of symptoms:

- 0 to 2 years: 11
- More than 2 to 5 years: 5
- More than 5 to 10 years: 9
- More than 10 to 20 years: 5
- More than 20 years: 2
- Undetermined: 27

Results of the treatment

- Very good:24 (40.6%)
- Good: 22 (37.3%)
- Fairly good:2 (3.4%)
- Failed: 11 (18.7%)

Treatment durations: 6 months to 6 years

Treatment stopped before 6 months: 14 patients:

- Improved: 9
- Failed: 5

Five schizophrenia

Treatment duration: 6 months to 4 years

Ancientness of symptoms: 2 to 9 years

Results of treatment

- Very good: 3
- Good: 1
- Failed: 1

Treatment stopped before 6 months: 4 patients:

- Good: 2
- Failed: 2

3 Borderline

Treatment durations: 6 months to 6 years

Ancientness of symptoms: 2 to 4 years

Result of treatment

- Very good: 1
- Good: 2

1 Delirium with relapses

Treatment duration: 3 years

Ancientness of symptoms: 3 and half years

Results of treatment: Very good

Ten children with agressivity; excitement

Treatment durations: 6 months to 2 years

Ancientness of symptoms: 1 month to 8 years

Results of treatment

- Very good: 9
- Good: 1

Treatment stopped before 6 months: 2 patients:

- Good: 1
- Failed: 1

One autistic child

Treatment duration: one year

Ancientness of symptoms: 12 years

Result of treatment: good

For schizophrenia, borderline, delirium children with aggressivity and autistic child: association with peripheral and central vascular problems.

CONCLUSION

All of Dr. Bottero's therapeutic results are confirmed since 1991 by Dr. Cecile Jadin of South Africa for more than 3000 CFS, and other psychopathological states (300) (Poster presentation at Sydney 98 CFS Conference, Australia) and also by Professor Nicolson (U.S.A.) using the same categories of antibiotics.

We have shown that Rickettsiae and Chlamydiae are probably caus-ative factors in many "psychopathologies."

Sometimes associated with other bacteria (Prof. Nicolson, CA, U.S.A.) and viral agents becoming reciprocally active (GJ 86 and JAD 84) and perhaps predetermining genetic factors; and with initial stress which is often observed.

Examples of pejorative associations: *Mycoplasma* and AIDS (LO Montagnier); Hepatitis B and the agent delta; Burkitt's lymphoma.

REFERENCES

BOT 87: P. Bottero. "Chronic psychopathologies associated with persistent rickett-siae and/or similar germs (chlamydiae)" Acta Mediterranea di Patologia Infettiva e Tropicale, 1987, *6* (3) (Proceedings of International Meeting "Rickettsiology: the present and the future," Palermo, Italy).

GAU 67: R. Gaudineau (Departement de Neuro-psychiatrie, Hôpital de. Bobo-Djou-lasso, Haute Volta) "En connection avec une probable étiologie rickettsienne dans les maladies du système nerveux" Bull. Soc. Path. Exot., 1967, *60*, 298-376.

GJ 86: P. Giroud et J.B. Jadin. "Les alliections superposées sont à la base des faillites de l'immunité" Arch. Inst. Pasteur, Tunis, 1986, *63*, 97-99.

GW58: S. Griesman et C. Wisseman. Bull. Soc. Path. Exot., 1958, *51*, 752.

JAD84: J.B. Jadin. "Relation entre protozaires, virus et bactéries" Revue de l'As-sociation Belge des technologues de Laboratoire, 1984, *11*, 9-22.

KKH93: Khin Khin Htwe and al. Prevalence of antibodies to *coxiella burnetii* in Japan. J. Clin. Microbiol., 1993 31(3): 732-740.

LM61: P. Loo et J. Menier. "Les rickettsies et nec-rickettsies en neuro-psychiatrie" Ann, de Médecine psychologique, 1961, *119* (2), 732-740.

LM 62: P. Loo et J. Menier. "Psychose intermittente et rickettsie" Ibid, 1962, *120* (1), 820-824.

MAS 63:A. Masbernard. "Les localisations neurologiques des rickettsioses" Bull. Soc. Path. Exot., 1963, 56, 714-740.

NL 19: C. Nicolle et C. Lebailly. "Les infections expérimentales inapparentes. Ex-emples tirés du typhus exanthématique" C.R. Acad. Sc, 1919, *168*, 800 and Arch. Inst. Pasteur, Tunis, *11*, 1-5.

FURTHER READING

P. Bottero. "Les formes psychiques des rickettsioses" Compte rendu des commu-nications consacrées aux rickettsioses et chlamydioses, 1986, Clinique Résidence du Parc, Marseille.

P. Giroud et M.L. Giroud. "Agglutination des rickettsies. Test de séro-protection et d'hypersensibilité cutanée." Bull. Soc. Path. Exot., 1944, *37*, 84.

P. Giroud, J.B. Jadin et M.C. Henry. "Au sujet des maladies rickettsiennes et celles dues aux agents proches in Europe Occidentale." Bull. des séances de l'Ac. Royale des Sc. d'outre-Mer, 1976, *3*, 420.

J.B. Jadin. "Les rickettsioses du Congo Belge et du Ruanda-Urundi." Thèse d'a-grégation de l'enseignement supérieur Ed. Nauwelaerts, Louvain (1951).

W.V. King. "Experimental transmission of Rocky Mountain Spotted Fever by means of the Tick." Preliminary Report, Pub. Health Rep., 1906, *21*, 863-864.

A. Pijper et C.B. Crocker. "Rickettsioses of South Afiica." South Afiica Med. J., 1938, *12*, 613-630.

H. Peron. "Thèse de diplôme d'étude approfondie de biologie cellulaire et molécul-aire: sérologie des rickettsioses (ELISA)" 1985, Département de Virologie, Centre Hospitalier Universitaire, Grenoble.

H.T. Ricketts. "The study of 'Rocky Mountain Spotted Fever' (Tick Fever) by means of animal inoculations." A preliminary communication J. Amer. Med. Ass., 1906, *47*, 33-36.

PROCEEDINGS OF INTERNATIONAL MEETING

The clinical and scientific basis of chronic fatigue syndrome "from myth towards management." The university of Newcastle, Sydney, Autralia, 11-12 February 1998.

Bottero Ph. "Rickettsiae and chlamydiae in patient psychopathology: A diagnostic and therapeutic report. (98 C.F.S. and 79 other)." Page 163.
Jadin C. C.F.S. "Rickettsiae infection. Presenting the result of 5 years of diagnostic and therapy."
Haier J., Nasralla M., Nicolson G.L. "Mycoplasmal infections in blood from patients with chronic fatigue syndrome, fibromyolgia syndrome or gulf war illness." Page 16.
Bernhard Liedtke, Bill Paspaliaris "Prevalence of *Coxiella burnetii* in Chronic Fatigue Syndrome" Poster presentation at Sydney, 1999, M.E./C.F.S. Conference, Australia. Page 25.

CLINICAL TREATMENT FOR RICKETTSIA AND CHLAMYDIA

Macrolides and cyclines are the two categories of antibiotics utilized. They can be used in conjunction/together.

The different macrolides are:

• Spiramycine	9 mg per day
• Clarithromycin	750 mg to 1 g per day
• Roxithromycin	450 mg per day
• Azithromycin	500 mg the first day and 250 mg per day during 4 days

The different cyclines are:

• Doxycycline	300 mg per day
• Tetracycline Chlorhydrate	2-3 g per day
• Minocycline	200-300 mg per day
• Lymecycline	226 mg × 6 per day
• Oxytetracycline	2-3 g per day

For children: Use the appropriate dose.

Macrolides and tetracyclins can be used in conjunction: 1/2 dose for each. Azithromycin must be used in conjunction with a cycline during ten days. For instance Minocyclines 200 mg per day or Tetracyclines 2 g per day or Doxycyclines 200 mg per day or Lymecyclines 226 mg × 4 per day.

The duration of the course of antibiotics is 10-12 days or more if the patient feels no distress.

One can observe an accentuation of symptoms when on antibiotics. This probably corresponds to a discharge of bacterial toxins and can be combated by anti-inflammatory medicines and warm bathes (perspiration).

Medicine for vascular system should be prescribed between the courses of antibiotics during 3 or 4 weeks:

• Naftidrofuryl (vasodilator)	400 mg per day
• Ginko Biloba (EGB 761) (vasodilator)	120 mg per day
• Trimetazidine (oxygenator)	40-60 mg per day
• Ifenprodil (vasodilator)	60 mg per day
• Pentoxifylline (vasodilator/oxygenator)	800 mg per day
• Piracetam (vasodilator)	2400 mg per day
• Buflomedil (vasodilator)	450 mg per day
• Papaverine Chlorhydrate	300 mg per day

These medicines can be utilised in children at an appropriate dose.

Combinations of vasodilators and oxygenators can be useful.

Anti-clotting agent/anti-platelet aggregating agent can be used (aspirin), perhaps heparin or anticoagulation medications? D. Berg, L.H. Berg, J. Couvaras (1). Don't forget that Rickettsiae and Chlamydiae are in the endothelium of blood vessels and could disturb endothelial functions. In case of low blood pressure use Heptaminol Chlorhydrate or Theodrenaline Chlorhydrate.

Chloroquine at a dose of 200 to 300 mg per day used in conjunction with antibiotics can increase the action of the antibiotics on *C. burnetti*.

In case of diarrhoea, use during antibiotics courses: *Saccharomyces boulardii*, 56.5 mg × 6 per day

The duration of treatment for chronic forms is one to two years minimum and much more in patients with a long history of the disease.

During the treatment some relapses occur but if the treatment is efficient they are less frequent.

The treatment must last 18 months before to conclude a failure.

Late relapses are always possible. They can be controlled by 2 or 3 courses of antibiotics. (Activation of latent infectious spots.)

Re-infestation from animals and insect vectors should be avoided at all cost.

The technique described above should be supplemented by use of hot baths (vasodilation and detoxification by perspiration) and advice on life hygiene. Don't forget that *Rickettsia* and *Coxiella burnetti* secrete vasoconstrictive toxins.

Advice to Be Followed Strictly

Techniques of hot bath:

- 1 pkt of seaweed per bath
- Duration: 20-30 minutes
- Temperature: 36 to 42°C
- Use the temperature which gives best perspiration but do not go any higher.
- Repeats: 2 to 3 times per week before taking another bath, the patient must have fully recovered from the previous one or else leave the next one untill full recovery from previous one has occured.
- After the bath–Do not dry yourself/(the patient), instead, wrap yourself/(the patient) in wool blanket and a quilt and lie in bed for 60 to 90 minutes.
- Drink a bowl of hot diuretic tea.
- The bath water must be kept at constant temperature and should reach mid-thorax.
- The bathroom and bedroom must be heated beforehand.

Life Hygiene:

Forbidden:

- Tobacco
- Alcohol

To be avoided:

- White wines
- Beer
- Fried foods
- Game birds
- Offals
- Game animals
- Prepared meats
- Animal fats
- Spices

To be encouraged:

- Sunflower oil
- Olive oil
- Green vegetables
- Fruits
- Complete cereals
- White meats
- Fish
- Lean red meat (all fat cut off)
- Polyvitamins

Avoid:

- Stationary position
- Stress
- Cold baths
- Extended stay in the sun

For massage treatments:

- Superfical massages aiming at stimulating circulation
- Physio-therapy in warm sea water
- No deep massages
- Respect delay of recuperation between each course of movements

Fight against constipation:

- Green vegetables
- Fruit

- Cereals
- Bran
- Grain/brown bread
- Prunes, etc.

Urinate more than 1.5 L per day.

Conjunction of Ampligen therapy and antibiotics could be very efficient because the immune defense against intra-cells small bacterias are near those induced by viral infections and interferon seems the most efficient mediator (2).

PS. Some patients react better to some treatments than others whether antibiotics or vaso-dilators/oxygenators are used–patients must be followed carefully.

PS. This treatment derives from the treatment of French military doctor General P. Legac (Deceased) for chronic rickettsiosis and chlamydiosis. Dr. Legac has made the first publication about association between chlamydiae and multiple sclerosis. (C.R. Académie des Sciences, Nov. 1966, Paris.)

1. D. Berg, L.H. Berg, J. Couvaras HEMEX Laboratories, IVF Phoenix. "Is C.F.S. due to an undefined hypercoagulable state brought on by immune activation of coagulation?" Poster Presentation at Sydney, 1999 M.E./C.F.S. Conference, Australia. Page 26.
2. C.W. Lapp, C.S. Voyles, P. Davis (U.S.A.) "Ampligen and chronic fatigue syndrome." Page 26. Proceeding of International Meeting, Sydney, Australia, 1998 (February). The clinical and scientific basis of chronic fatigue syndrome.

Chronic Psychopathologies Associated with Persistent Rickettsiae and/or Similar Germs (Chlamydiae)

Philippe Bottero, MD

SUMMARY. For 60 cases of diseases that are called "Psychic" associated with persistent rickettsiae; we have: 55 good and excellent result, 5 failure, but we still have to wait a confirmation in course of time for many patients.

KEYWORDS. *Rickettsia, Chlamydia*

I would like to begin by describing the framework and setting, the direction and aim of my intervention.

It consists of medical practitioner in contact with his patients, who while treating them, records a considerable improvement of the pathological symptoms in a great majority of cases over a variable period.

Somewhat scholastic arguments concerning the value or non-value a serologic reaction, which seems in actual fact to depend on the antigenic quality of the strains used, must be relativised.

Philippe Bottero is Faculté de Médecine, Paris, France, 10 Avenue Henri Rochier 26110 Nyons, France (E-mail: p.botter@caramail.com).

This article is reprinted with permission from *Acta Mediterranea di Patologia Infettiva e Tropicale*, 1987, 6 (3):339-345.

[Haworth co-indexing entry note]: "Chronic Psychopathologies Associated with Persistent Rickettsiae and/or Similar Germs (Chlamydiae)." Bottero, Philippe. Co-published simultaneously in *Journal of Chronic Fatigue Syndrome* (The Haworth Medical Press, an imprint of The Haworth Press, Inc.) Vol. 6, No. 3/4, 2000, pp. 163-170; and: *Chronic Fatigue Syndrome: Critical Reviews and Clinical Advances* (ed: Kenny De Meirleir, and Roberto Patarca-Montero) The Haworth Medical Press, an imprint of The Haworth Press, Inc., 2000, pp. 163-170.

In point of fact a serologic reaction assumes full value when it is confronted on the one hand with the symptomatology and on the other hand with the development under treatment and finally with its dynamic aspect which shows in all our cases a significant variation in the antibody titres from one examination to another or over a longer period with intermittent almost constant negativation.

To be sure, we have not tested the therapeutic according to the terms of the modalities in force; but most of our patients have done so for a number of months or years in pathology, even going back decades, and have tried multiple therapeutics without success and have thus in my opinion exhausted every "Placebo" effect possible.

Our results are at last beginning to be cross-checked and confirmed by French doctors whom we have trained.

The symptoms I observed were in part dealt with previously by medical practioners in the 1960s who had already opened the gateway of rickettsial psychopathology.

To these foundations, I have added my own stone to the edifice.

In a like manner it also rests with the clinician with his sense of observation to put forth sufficiently convincing and convergent arguments in order that the university authorities, with the means they have at their disposal, provide absolute proof of what we are proposing.

It would be interesting to verify if a certain number of our seropositive cases are also seropositive vis-à-vis the Borrelioses, notably the *Borrelia burgdorferi*, whose epidemiology is close, which is responsible for the Lyme disease whose delayed chronic manifestations can be neuropsychic.

I thank Doctor-General Legac (Médecin des Hôpitaux), who demonstrated the considerable role of rickettsiae in the origin of multiple schlerosis; Professor Jadin of the Institute of Tropical Medicine of Anvers who trained me in the field of rickettsiae; Professor Henri Baruk of the Academy of Medicine of Paris, a great figure of French organic psychiatry, whose broadness of mind has allowed me to become acquainted with the vast field of psychopathology presumed "Rickettsial" and to embark on a fruitful collaboration.

Finally I will add that numerous positive seroreactions in the Giroud microagglutination test have been confirmed by the reaction of immunofluorescence, both by Professor Jadin and in a French laboratory; the correlation has been excellent, not so much as on the strains of virus, as on the seropositivity; and in ELISA on 28 sera (C. Perron, Grenoble, 1985). Twenty-two sera have been tested by microagglutionation on a Giroud slope by Professor Jadin of the Institute of Tropical Medicine of Anvers. This test consists of strains propagated in embryonated eggs and by immunofluorescence (IF) in a French laboratory working on strains prepared by the Merieux Laboratories (France).

Seven of the sera were tested in multiple on the same day.

A total of 22:22 were revealed positive in microaglutination and 20:22 positive in IF with significant titres.

Here are 15 sera tested at different dates:

GAU	30.10.86	R. prowazeki	+++	1/320	
		R. mooseri	+++	1/160	
	30.10.86	R. conori		1/40	(IFI)
RIC	Feb. 87	R. mooseri	++++	1/160	
	25.5.87	R. conori		1/40	(IFI)
LAP	Oct. 86	R. conori	++++	1/160	
	13.3.87	R. mooseri		1/40	(IFI)
		R. conori		1/40	
BOU	Nov. 86	R. mooseri	+++	1/160	
		R. burnetti	(II) ++++	1/20	
	13.3.87	R. conori		1/80	(IFI)
		R. mooseri		1/40	
MAR	5.6.87	R. conori		1/40	(IFI)
		R. mooseri		1/40	
	2.2.87	R. mooseri	++++	1/160	
		R. burnetti	(II) ++++	1/20	
GAY	29.6.87	R. conori		1/40	(IFI)
		C. burnetti		1/160	
	10.4.87	R. mooseri	++++	1/160	
		E. conori	+++	1/160	
		C. burnetti	(II) ++++	1/20	
CUC	1.7.87	R. conori		1/40	(IFI)
	22.4.87	R. prowazecki	+++	1/320	
	microaggl.	R. mooseri	++++	1/160	
	tintation	C. burnetti	(II) +++	1/20	
	(Giroud)				

EVE	29.5.87	*R. conori*		1/40	} (IFI)
		R. mooseri		1/40	
	19.3.87	*R. prowazecki*	+++	1/320	
		R. mooseri	++++	1/160	
		C. burnetti	(II) ++++	1/20	
DUC	23.6.87	*R. conori*		1/40	(IFI)
		C. burnetti		1/80	
	16.4.86	*R. mooseri*	++++	1/160	
		R. conori	+++	1/160	
FRE	11.12.86	*R. conori*		1/160	} (IFI)
		R. mooseri		1/40	
	6.6.86	*R. mooseri*	++++	1/160	
BER L.	24.5.85	*R. mooseri*	++++	1/160	
		R. conori	+++	1/160	
	17.12.86	*R. conori*		1/160	} (IFI)
		R. mooseri		1/40	
BER C.	11.12.86	*R. conori*	Negative		(IFI)
		C. burnetti			
		R. mooseri			
	Nov. 85	*R. mooseri*	++++	1/160	
MOR	23.7.86	*R. conori*		1/320	} (IFI)
		R. mooseri		1/80	
		C. burnetti	negative		
	29.6.86	*R. mooseri*	++++	1/160	
GUI	30.1.87	*R. mooseri*	++++	1/160	
		C. burnetti	(II) ++++	1/20	
	27.4.87	*R. conori*		1/40	(IFI)
FLA	20.11.86	*R. prowazecki*	++++	1/320	
		R. mooseri	++++	1/160	
		R. conori	++++	1/160	
		C. burnetti	(II) ++++	1/20	
	3.6.87	*R. conori*		1/160	} (IFI)
		R. mooseri		1/40	

*   *   *

Here are the 7 sera tested on the same day:

EST	*R. conori*	1/40	(IFI)	*R. mooseri*	+++	1/160
FER	Negative		(IFI)	*R. mooseri*	+++	1/160
VAL	*R. conori*	1/40	(IFI)	*R. conori*	++++	1/160

POR	R. conori	1/80⎱	(IFI)	R. mooseri	++++	1/160
	R. mooseri	1/40⎰		C. burnetti	++++	1/20
GAL	R. conori	1/80	(IFI)	R. mooseri	++++	1/160
				R. prowazecki	+++	1/320
LET	R. conori	1/40	(IFI)	R. mooseri	+++	1/160
				R. conori	++++	1/160
DEI	R. conori	1/40	(IFI)	R. prowazecki	++++	1/320
				R. mooseri	++++	1/160
				R. conori	+++++	1/160

As regards the sera tested in ELISA, they are multiple schlerosis sera all positive in microagglutination (Giroud) which are all revealed positive in ELISA vis-à-vis *R. conori* (cultivated on embyonated eggs; Professor Jadin) with presence of Ig6 in 81.5% of cases, and presence of IgM in 82% of cases.

This work was carried out in the Virology Department of C.H.U. of Grenoble (France) (Perron H. 1985).

The neuropsychic impact is almost constant in acute rickettsiae or even chronic in the instance of extra-neurological foci owing to the fact that the properties of the rickettsial toxins, which are vaso-constrictive and demylinising; and which are discharged into the circulatory stream (experiment by Levaditi) and also due to the fact of the great sensitivity of nerve cells to anoxia and by the slight possibility of their regeneration.

The neuropsychopathological manifestations of acute rickettsiae have been described by numerous writers, including Porot as early as 1909 for the typhus epidemic: deranged state at times manic-depressive tonality, deliria with onirism, ambulatory automatisms, at times suicidal impulses (jumping from window), quite unusual disorders of the body scheme and of consciousness, at time preluding stupor and coma.

These disorders can open up the clinical scene and pose diagnostic difficulties even in an epidemic milieu and can be revelatory (typhus epidemic in Serbia during the World War I).

Generally regressive, they are able to develop in only one case out of a hundred, according to Guttman, towards a deranged or chonic psychotic state, either immediately following on the acute episode or which a delayed appearance, being able to last for more than ten years.

The present world-wide spreading of richettsiae, their tendancy to chronicity directly after an acute episode or unapparent primary or secondary infection after a varied period of latency, as numerous authors have recorded after Charles Nicolle and have shown the clinical and epidemiological importance of the long survival of the virulent rickettsiae in their haunts in the reticuloendothelium and vascular linings, allows one to think that a certain number of chronic psychopathological and psychiatric pictures can claim this etiology: chronic Richettsial vascular encephalitis.

Moreover certain authors incline towards this possible etiology: Gaudineau R. (Department of Neuropsychiatry, Hospital of Bobo-Dioulasso, Upper Volta), in connection with a probable rickettsaie etiology of the impairment of nervous system: (*Bull. Sco. De Pathologie Exotique*, 1967, 298-376); Loo P. and Menier J., "Les Rickettsies et neorickettsies en neuro-psychiatrie" (*Ann. De Médécine Psychologique*, 1967, 119 2, 732); Loo P. and Menier J., "Psychose intermittente et rickettsies" (Ibid., 1962, 120, 1, 820), and a great many other authors.

How is one to arrive at a diagnostic etiology of psychopathic and chronic psychiatric states, all the more difficult as the form becomes more focalised? There I base myself upon my clinical experience and for the majority of therapeutic cases: going from certain syndromes know as "tetanic spasmophile" associated with psychic disturbances, to certain nervous depressions, passing by the clinical pictures of psychoneurotic, hypochondriac or hysterical children in order to terminate with the psychotic pictures, and the schizophrenic and delirious aspect.

A certain number of arguments—epidemiological, clinical, serological, evolutive and therapeutic—must be regrouped.

Epidemiological: Tick bites, contacts with animals of every type, exposed professions, travels to regions of the endemic disease, holidays on farms, consumption of raw milk: facts which are less convincing at present in view of the multiplicity of domestic animals, trips abroad, holidays in the country (farm, camping, etc.).

Clinical: It is to be noted that among all the forms there are common symptoms which are quite regularly re-encountered: frequent first appearance after either psychic or physical traumatism (or both), straight away or at later date.

Several cases within siblings (veritable families of rickettsia exist):

development in sudden bouts or complete remisssions, at least at the outset, notably at changes of season and with atmospheric pressure or after stress in the broad sense of the term; bout of fever (inconstant), aggressivity, irritability; depression capable of leading to suicide, attraction by space (temptation to jump from heights), hypersensitivity to noise, light, smell, vertigo or false vertigo, loss of balance, occasional weakness of the knees resulting in their collapsing, veritable drop attacks, dropping of objects, phenomena of moving spots before the eyes, the seeing of bright lights or shapes, visual eclipses, double or triple vision, visual or auditory hallucinations, delusions of persecution, ambulatory automatism, frenzied convictions, numbness and tingling sensation of the extremities, cold and stiff with cyanosis, vasomotor syndromes able to reach the point of Raynaud's disease, hypersensibility of the extremities to cold, hot flushes, headache (frequent), spontaneous bruising (vascular fragility), muscular cramps, myalgias contractions of the hands, erratic even congestive and febrile arthralgia, dorsal aches, electric discharges, thoracic oppressions with anxiety, digestive troubles (frequent), profound asthenia (more or less permanent), tachycardiac attacks, palpitations, lipothymic tendancy notably on changes of position up to the point of losing consciousness, hypertension, behavioural instability, impression of an imaginary presence, buzzing of the ears, decline in hearing, loss of memory and intellectual concentration, all signs varying from one day to another and associated differently during the day.

Finally a multiplicity of doctors consulted and medicines tried without result.

The most frequent clinical signs to be found are:

- malaise on changing position;
- vertigo (real or false);
- paresthesis of the extremities;
- vaso-motors flushes;
- drop in temperature of the extremities (permanent or intermittent) with hypersensitivity to cold;
- distress, tachycardiac attacks, depression, aggressivity;
- troubles of intellectual concentration;
- phenomena of seeing spots before the eyes;
- digestive troubles of colitic type; and
- asthenia with psychasthenia.

Serological: Positivity of the microagglutination reaction to often highly raised titres, immediatly or after reactivation during treatment: the murine and boutonneuse antigens being more often found, followed by a considerable variation of antibody titres, from one examination to the other or at longer intervals, and intermittent practically constant total negativation, often, but not always, corresponding to the periods of remission.

Therapeutic: Favourable development very frequent under treatment, either immediatly or at a secondary stage, in the knowledge that the treatment will be very long, several years in chronic forms of longstanding. Besides, the first courses of antibiotic treatments often produce a reactivation of the disorders.

With respect to schizophrenia, out of four cases: 100% positive: one borderline case under treatment with very favourable development after two and half years; finally five cases of syndromes of delirium with relapses, positive.

For five out of these six cases, there are certain disorders previously cited associated with an initial Raynaud syndrome.

Two cases of schizophrenia belonging to the same family, each member of which excepting the father, namely the mother and one sister, present anxiety–depressive disorders and symptoms associated with a similar circulatory aspect.

Index

Academy of Medicine of Paris, 164
Acquired immuno-deficiency
        syndrome (AIDS), 32-34,42
Activation-induced cell death, 41-50
AIDS. *See* Acquired
        immuno-deficiency
        syndrome (AIDS)
ALS. *See* Amyotropic lateral sclerosis
        (ALS)
Alzheimer's disease, 83-84
Amyotropic lateral sclerosis (ALS),
        33-34
Antibiotics as clinical treatments,
        34-36,157-161
Arthritis, rheumatoid. *See* Rheumatoid
        arthritis (RA)

Bacteria
        Chlamydiae. See
                Chlamydiae-related diseases
        microbiology of chronic fatigue
                syndrome (CFS), 10-11
        Rickettsiae. See Rickettsial-related
                diseases
        specific bacteria associated with
                fatigue-related diseases,
                23-39,134-136,147-161,
                164-167
Baraniuk, J.N., 81
Barker, E., 74,75,76
Barker, L., 19
Baruk, H., 164
Basal ganglia and neurological
        dysfunction, 51-68
Bastien, S., 12,13
Beard, G., 52
Behan, P.O., 51-68
Bennett, A.L., 89,91

Bervoets, K., 17
Biochemistry of chronic fatigue
        syndrome (CFS), 4-8,17-18
Biorhythms of fatigue and chronic
        fatigue syndrome (CFS)
        introduction to, 109-110
        studies of (results), 110-113
        studies of (subjects and methods),
                110
Blanchard, A., 33
Blood pressure, high. *See*
                Cardiovascular-related
                diseases
Boelyn, A., 52
Borish, L., 81
Borok, G., 81
Borysiewicz, L.K., 72, 78
Bottero, P., 11,13,19,134,147-161,
        163-170
Brostoff, J., 8,9
Bruno, R.L., 62
Buchwald, D., 71,72,78,87,89,90
Butt, H., 5,10,11

Cabane, J., 13,109-116
Caligiuri, M., 75
Cancer and cancer-related diseases,
        142
Cannon, J.G., 84
Cardiovascular-related diseases,
        133,135f,140-141
Carter, W., 15
CFS. *See* Chronic fatigue syndrome
                (CFS), general information
                about
CFS/ME. *See* Myalgic
                encephalomyelitis (ME)
Chao, C.C., 89